Gluten-Free Vegan Cookbook

1500 Days of Delicious, Super Easy Recipes and Meal Plans to Transform Your Health and Boost Energy Levels

DR LANA BROWN, RN

Copyright Page

© 2024 by Dr. Lana Brown.

Table of Contents

CHAPTER I

THE GLUTEN-FREE VEGAN LIFESTYLE

Gluten is a family of proteins found in grains, including wheat, rye, spelt, and barley.

Of the gluten-containing grains, wheat is by far the most common, Glutenin and gliadin are the two main proteins in gluten. Gliadin is responsible for most of the adverse health effects of gluten.

When flour mixes with water, the gluten proteins form a sticky network that has a glue-like consistency.

This glue-like property makes the dough elastic and gives bread the ability to rise during baking. It also provides a chewy, satisfying texture.

Interestingly, the name gluten derives from this glue-like property of wet dough.

Most people can tolerate gluten with no adverse effects. However, it can cause problems for people with certain health conditions.

Intolerance vs. sensitivity

Digestive discomfort is the most common indication of gluten intolerance. The person may also have anemia or trouble gaining weight.

To determine the cause of the discomfort, people can ask their doctor to check for celiac disease first.

There are two main ways to determine if a person has celiac disease:

- **Blood tests:** Several blood tests screen for antibodies. A common one is the tTG-IgA test. If that is positive, the doctor may recommend a tissue biopsy to confirm the results.

- **Biopsy from small intestine**: A health professional takes a small tissue sample from the small intestine, which a lab analyzes for damage.

A person should undertake both of the above tests while following a gluten-containing diet. Performing the blood test while on a gluten-free diet will yield a false negative. This is because there is no gluten in the system to trigger antibody production.

If a person thinks they may have celiac disease, they should consult their doctor before trying a gluten-free diet.

If the person does not have celiac disease, the best way to find out if they are sensitive to gluten is to follow a strict gluten-free diet for a few weeks to see if symptoms improve.

Then, they will need to introduce gluten back into their diet to see if their symptoms return.

If the person's symptoms do not improve on a gluten-free diet and do not get worse when they reintroduce gluten, then the cause is probably something other than gluten.

A gluten-free diet test is not a definite way to diagnose the issue, and people should not try this on their own. If a person suspects they may have a problem, they should seek guidance from a healthcare professional who can test for celiac disease or allergies.

Celiac Disease

Celiac disease is an illness caused by an immune reaction to eating gluten. If you have celiac disease, eating gluten triggers an immune response to the gluten protein in your small intestine. Over time, this reaction damages your small intestine's lining and prevents it from absorbing nutrients, a condition called malabsorption.

The intestinal damage often causes symptoms such as diarrhea, fatigue, weight loss, bloating or anemia. It also can lead to serious complications if it is not managed or treated. In children, malabsorption can affect growth and development in addition to gastrointestinal symptoms.

There's no definite cure for celiac disease. But for most people, following a strict gluten-free diet can help manage symptoms and help the intestines heal.

Symptoms

The symptoms of celiac disease can vary greatly. They also may be different in children and adults. Digestive symptoms for adults include:

• Diarrhea.

• Fatigue.

• Weight loss.

• Bloating and gas.

• Abdominal pain.

• Nausea and vomiting.

• Constipation.

However, more than half the adults with celiac disease have symptoms that are not related to the digestive system, including:

• Anemia, usually from iron deficiency due to decreased iron absorption.

• Loss of bone density, called osteoporosis, or softening of bones, called osteomalacia.

• Itchy, blistery skin rash, called dermatitis herpetiformis.

• Mouth ulcers.

• Headaches and fatigue.

• Nervous system injury, including numbness and tingling in the feet and hands, possible problems with balance, and cognitive impairment.

• Joint pain.

• Reduced functioning of the spleen, known as hyposplenism.

• Elevated liver enzymes.

Children

Children with celiac disease are more likely than adults to have digestive problems, including:

• Nausea and vomiting.

• Chronic diarrhea.

• Swollen belly.

• Constipation.

• Gas.

• Pale, foul-smelling stools.

The inability to absorb nutrients might result in:

• Failure to thrive for infants.

• Damage to tooth enamel.

• Weight loss.

• Anemia.

• Irritability.

• Short stature.

• Delayed puberty.

• Neurological symptoms, including attention-deficit/hyperactivity disorder (ADHD), learning disabilities, headaches, lack of muscle coordination and seizures.

Causes

Your genes, combined with eating foods with gluten and other factors, can contribute to celiac disease. However, the precise cause isn't known. Infant-feeding practices, gastrointestinal infections and gut bacteria may contribute, but these causes have not been proved. Sometimes celiac disease becomes active after surgery, pregnancy, childbirth, viral infection or severe emotional stress.

When the body's immune system overreacts to gluten in food, the reaction damages the tiny, hairlike projections, called villi, which line the small intestine. Villi absorb vitamins, minerals and other nutrients from the food you eat. If your villi are damaged, you can't get enough nutrients, no matter how much you eat.

Risk factors

Celiac disease tends to be more common in people who have:

• A family member with celiac disease or dermatitis herpetiformis.

• Type 1 diabetes.

• Down syndrome, William syndrome or Turner syndrome.

• Autoimmune thyroid disease.

• Microscopic colitis.

• Addison's disease.

Complications

Celiac disease that is not treated can lead to:

• **Malnutrition.** This occurs if your small intestine can't absorb enough nutrients. Malnutrition can lead to anemia and weight loss. In children, malnutrition can cause slow growth and short stature.

• **Bone weakening.** In children, malabsorption of calcium and vitamin D can lead to a softening of the bone, called osteomalacia or rickets. In adults, it can lead to a loss of bone density, called osteopenia or osteoporosis.

• **Infertility and miscarriage.** Malabsorption of calcium and vitamin D can contribute to reproductive issues.

• **Lactose intolerance**. Damage to your small intestine might cause you abdominal pain and diarrhea after eating or drinking dairy products that contain lactose. Once your intestine has healed, you might be able to tolerate dairy products again.

• **Cancer.** People with celiac disease who don't maintain a gluten-free diet have a greater risk of developing several forms of cancer, including intestinal lymphoma and small bowel cancer.

• **Nervous system conditions.** Some people with celiac disease can develop conditions such as seizures or a disease of the nerves to the hands and feet, called peripheral neuropathy.

Nonresponsive celiac disease

Some people with celiac disease don't respond to what they consider to be a gluten-free diet. Nonresponsive celiac disease is often due to contamination of the diet with gluten. Working with a dietitian can help you learn how to avoid all gluten.

People with nonresponsive celiac disease might have:

• Bacterial overgrowth in the small intestine.

• Microscopic colitis.

• Poor pancreas function, known as pancreatic insufficiency.

• Irritable bowel syndrome.

• Difficulty digesting sugar found in dairy products (lactose), table sugar (sucrose), or a type of sugar found in honey and fruits (fructose).

• Truly refractory celiac disease that is not responding to a gluten-free diet.

Refractory celiac disease

In rare instances, the intestinal injury of celiac disease doesn't respond to a strict gluten-free diet. This is known as refractory celiac disease. If you still have symptoms after following a gluten-free diet for 6 months to 1 year, you should talk to your health care team to see if you need further testing to look for explanations for your symptoms.

Dermatitis herpetiformis

Gluten intolerance can cause this blistery skin disease. The rash usually occurs on the elbows, knees, torso, scalp or buttocks. This condition is often associated with changes to the lining of the small intestine identical to those of celiac disease, but the skin condition might not cause digestive symptoms.

Health care professionals treat dermatitis herpetiformis with a gluten-free diet or medicine, or both, to control the rash.

Diagnosis

Many people with celiac disease don't know they have it. Two blood tests can help diagnose it:

• Serology testing looks for antibodies in your blood. Elevated levels of certain antibody proteins indicate an immune reaction to gluten.

• Genetic testing for human leukocyte antigens (HLA-DQ2 and HLA-DQ8) can be used to rule out celiac disease.

It's important to be tested for celiac disease before trying a gluten-free diet. Eliminating gluten from your diet might make the results of blood tests appear in the standard range.

If the results of these tests indicate celiac disease, one of the following tests will likely be ordered:

• **Endoscopy.** This test uses a long tube with a tiny camera that's put into your mouth and passed down your throat. The camera enables the practitioner to view your small intestine and take a small tissue sample, called a biopsy, to analyze for damage to the villi.

• **Capsule endoscopy.** This test uses a tiny wireless camera to take pictures of your entire small intestine. The camera sits inside a vitamin-sized capsule, which you swallow. As the capsule travels through your digestive tract, the camera takes thousands of pictures that are transmitted to a recorder. This test is used in some situations where an exam of the entire or end of the small intestine is desired.

If you might have dermatitis herpetiformis, your health care professional may take a small sample of skin tissue to examine under a microscope.

If you're diagnosed with celiac disease, additional testing may be recommended to check your nutritional status. This includes levels of vitamins A, B-12, D and E, as well as mineral levels, hemoglobin and liver enzymes. Your bone health also may be checked with a bone density scan.

Treatment

A strict, lifelong gluten-free diet is the only way to manage celiac disease. Besides wheat, foods that contain gluten include:

• Barley.

• Bulgur.

• Durum.

• Farina.

• Graham flour.

• Malt.

• Rye.

• Semolina.

• Spelt (a form of wheat).

• Triticale.

A dietitian who works with people with celiac disease can help you plan a healthy gluten-free diet. Even trace amounts of gluten in your diet can be damaging, even if they don't cause symptoms.

Gluten can be hidden in foods, medicines and nonfood products, including:

• Modified food starch, preservatives and food stabilizers.

• Prescription and over-the-counter medications.

• Vitamin and mineral supplements.

• Herbal and nutritional supplements.

• Lipstick products.

• Toothpaste and mouthwash.

• Communion wafers.

• Envelope and stamp glue.

• Play dough.

• Certain makeup products.

Removing gluten from your diet will typically reduce inflammation in your small intestine, causing you to feel better and eventually heal. Children tend to heal more quickly than adults.

Vitamin and mineral supplements

If your anemia or nutritional deficiencies are severe, supplements may be recommended, including:

• Copper.

• Folic acid.

• Iron.

• Vitamin B-12.

• Vitamin D.

• Vitamin K.

• Zinc.

Vitamins and supplements are usually taken in pill form. If your digestive tract has trouble absorbing vitamins, you might be able to get them by injection.

Follow-up care

Medical follow-up at regular intervals can ensure that your symptoms have responded to a gluten-free diet. Your health care team may monitor your response with blood tests. Nutritional markers also are checked regularly.

For most people with celiac disease, eating a gluten-free diet allows the small intestine to heal. For children, that usually takes 3 to 6 months. For adults, complete healing might take several years.

If you continue to have symptoms or if symptoms recur, you might need an endoscopy with biopsies to determine whether your intestine has healed.

Medications to control intestinal inflammation

If your small intestine is severely damaged or you have refractory celiac disease, steroids may be recommended to control inflammation. Steroids can ease severe symptoms of celiac disease while the intestine heals.

Other drugs, such as azathioprine (Azasan, Imuran) or budesonide (Entocort EC, Uceris), might be used.

Treating dermatitis herpetiformis

If you have this skin rash, a medicine called dapsone may be recommended in addition to a gluten-free diet. Dapsone is taken by mouth. If you take dapsone, you'll need regular blood tests to check for side effects.

Refractory celiac disease

With refractory celiac disease, the small intestine doesn't heal. Refractory celiac disease can be quite serious, and there is currently no proven treatment. If you have refractory celiac disease, you may want to seek medical care at a specialized center.

Lifestyle and home remedies

If you've been diagnosed with celiac disease, you'll need to avoid all foods that contain gluten. Ask your health care team for a referral to a dietitian, who can help you plan a healthy gluten-free diet.

Read labels

Avoid packaged foods unless they're labeled as gluten-free or have no gluten-containing ingredients, including emulsifiers and stabilizers that can contain gluten. In addition to cereals, pastas and baked goods, other packaged foods that can contain gluten include:

• Beers, lagers, ales and malt vinegars.

• Candies.

• Gravies.

• Imitation meats or seafood.

• Processed luncheon meats.

• Rice mixes.

• Salad dressings and sauces, including soy sauce.

• Seasoned snack foods, such as tortilla and potato chips.

• Seitan.

• Self-basting poultry.

• Soups.

Pure oats aren't harmful for most people with celiac disease, but oats can be contaminated by wheat during growing and processing. Ask your health care team if you can try eating small amounts of pure oat products.

Allowed foods

Many basic foods are allowed in a gluten-free diet, including:

• Eggs.

• Fresh meats, fish and poultry that aren't breaded, batter-coated or marinated.

• Fruits.

• Lentils.

• Most dairy products, unless they make your symptoms worse.

• Nuts.

• Potatoes.

• Vegetables.

• Wine and distilled liquors, ciders and spirits.

Grains and starches allowed in a gluten-free diet include:

• Amaranth.

• Buckwheat.

• Corn.

• Cornmeal.

• Gluten-free flours (rice, soy, corn, potato, bean).

• Pure corn tortillas.

• Quinoa.

• Rice.

• Tapioca.

• Wild rice.

Coping and support

It can be difficult, and stressful, to follow a completely gluten-free diet. Here are some ways to help you cope and to feel more in control.

• **Get educated and teach family and friends.** They can support your efforts in dealing with the disease.

• **Follow your health care professional's recommendations.** It's critical to eliminate all gluten from your diet.

• **Find a support group.** You might find comfort in sharing your struggles with people who face similar challenges. Organizations such as the Celiac Disease Foundation, Gluten Intolerance Group, the National Celiac Association and Beyond Celiac can help put you in touch with others who share your challenges.

The Principles of Veganism: What It Means to Be Vegan

Veganism, the theory or practice of abstaining from the consumption and use of animal products. While some vegans avoid only animal-derived food, many others also exclude any items that use animals as ingredients or for testing. These prohibited products can range from clothing (e.g., leather) to makeup. Dietary veganism differs from vegetarianism in that vegetarians may choose to consume some animal-derived foods such as milk, eggs, and honey on the grounds that animals do not need to be slaughtered to obtain these products. Veganism is motivated by a variety of reasons, including personal health, animal rights, environmentalism, and ethics. It is generally practiced less as a dietary preference and more as a lifestyle choice and form of activism.

The origins of veganism

The word "vegan" was coined in the UK in the 20th century, but its ideals date back thousands of years.

In 1944, a vegetarian named Donald Watson, who also chose not to eat dairy, decided that there should be a word to depict people like himself. He landed on "vegan," as it contained the first three and last two letters of "vegetarian." In 1949, Leslie J Cross (the former vice president of the Vegan Society), defined veganism as "the principle of the emancipation of animals from exploitation by man."

But Watson and Cross were by no means the first to take a stance against animal exploitation. Many people mistakenly believe that veganism is a predominantly white and western way of living. But its origins date back thousands of years to a number of different cultures across the world.

Siddhārtha Gautama (also known as the Buddha) endorsed vegetarianism to his followers when he lived in the 5th or 6th century BC. In the same period of time, the religions of Hinduism and

Jainism, both of which are still prominent today, were advocating for meat-free diets.

In 500 BC, Greek philosopher and mathematician Pythagoras of Samo endorsed kindness toward animals, and chose not to eat them. He also taught this ethical stance to his followers.

According to the latest definition from the Vegan Society, veganism is "a philosophy and way of living which seeks to exclude — as far as is possible and practicable — all forms of exploitation of, and cruelty to, animals for food, clothing, or any other purposes."

Many people use the term "vegan" to refer exclusively to diet. However, by this latest definition, veganism extends beyond eating a plant-based diet.

Those who identify as vegans typically aim to exclude animal exploitation or cruelty in all aspects of their lives, including the clothes they wear, the cosmetics they use, and the leisure activities they take part in.

As a result, many vegans avoid purchasing wool coats, leather furniture, or down pillows and comforters. They may also opt to visit animal sanctuaries instead of going to zoos, the circus, or animal petting farms.

Philosophy, ethics, and activism

Unlike most dietary choices, veganism is more often seen as a philosophical proposition, an ethical choice, and a form of individual activism that aims to have a global impact. Philosophers from Pythagoras to Peter Singer, the author of such books as *Animal Liberation* (1975), have argued that humans do not have the right to exploit or inflict suffering on animals and that such exploitation is unethical. Similarly, followers of Hinduism, Jainism, and Buddhism may become vegetarian or vegan on the basis of ahimsa, the ethical principle of not causing harm to any living being.

The modern vegan movement is tied to the formation of the Vegan Society in 1944. While initially focused mainly on animal rights, vegan activism more recently has also focused on the relationship between the consumption and use of animal products and climate change. On a global level, intensive animal farming has been shown to be a major contributor of the greenhouse gases causing global warming. On local levels, intensive animal farms and feedlots can pollute air and water in their immediate locations. The rise in livestock production for food has led to a dramatic increase in deforestation, especially in the Amazon region. Author Jonathan Safran Foer, who explored the ethics of meat consumption in his book *Eating Animals* (2009), wrote about the effects of animal consumption on climate change in his book *We Are the Weather: Saving the Planet Begins at Breakfast* (2019). In addition, activists have accused factory farming of committing animal cruelty.

Why do people go vegan?

People generally choose to avoid animal products for one or more of the following reasons.

Ethics

Ethical vegans strongly believe that all creatures have a right to life and freedom.

They view all animals as conscious beings that, just like humans, wish to avoid pain and suffering.

Because of this, ethical vegans are opposed to killing an animal in order to eat its flesh or wear its fur or skin.

Vegans are also opposed to the psychological and physical stress that animals may endure as a result of modern farming practices — for instance, the small pens or cages that animals typically live in and rarely leave between their birth and slaughter.

However, for ethical vegans, this sentiment extends beyond the cruelty of modern farming practices.

That's because vegans are opposed to consuming products that heavily rely on the killing of other animals — especially because alternatives are available.

This includes the slaughter of calves that are considered surplus in the dairy industry, or the culling of 1-day-old male chicks that is common in egg production.

Moreover, ethical vegans generally believe that animals' milk, eggs, honey, silk, and wool are not for humans to exploit, regardless of the living conditions afforded to the exploited animals.

This is why ethical vegans remain opposed to drinking an animal's milk, eating its eggs, or wearing its wool, even in cases where the animals are free-roaming or pasture-fed.

Health

Some people choose a vegan diet for its potential health benefits.

Diets high in meat — especially red meat — have been linked to cancer, heart disease, and type 2 diabetes.

On the other hand, plant-based diets have been linked to a lower risk of developing or prematurely dying from these diseases.

Lowering your intake of animal products in favor of more plant-based options may also improve your digestion and reduce your risk of Alzheimer's disease.

A vegan diet can also help minimize the side effects linked to the antibiotics and hormones used in modern animal agriculture.

Finally, vegan diets appear to be especially effective at helping people lose unwanted weight. Several studies link a vegan diet to a lower likelihood of obesity.

However, if you're on a vegan diet, you may consume less of certain nutrients. That's why planning is especially important.

Consider speaking with a healthcare professional, such as a doctor or registered dietitian, to plan a vegan diet that will help you get the nutrients you need.

Vegan diets tend to be low in these nutrients:

• Vitamin B12

• Vitamin D

• Calcium

• Zinc

• Iodine

• Selenium

People on vegan diets sometimes take supplements to provide nutrients they may not get enough of in their diet.

Environment

People may also choose to avoid animal products in an attempt to limit their environmental impact.

According to recent data, animal agriculture heavily contributes to greenhouse gas emissions (GHGEs), which cause climate change.

Meat eaters are thought to be responsible for 2–2.5 times more GHGEs than people following a vegan diet. This number is based on self-reported dietary patterns in the U.K.

Ruminant animals, such as cattle, sheep, and goats, appear to emit the largest amount of greenhouse gases per gram of protein they deliver. Therefore, diets that reduce or totally eliminate dairy also produce significantly fewer GHGEs.

One study suggests that a vegetarian diet produces 33% fewer GHGEs than a meat-containing standard American diet offering the same amount of calories.

A vegan diet has an even smaller environmental impact, producing about 53% fewer GHGEs than a calorie-matched meat-containing diet.

A large proportion of the plant protein currently being produced is used to feed animals rather than humans. Because of this, production of an animal-heavy diet requires use of more of the earth's resources than production of a plant-based diet.

For instance, producing animal protein requires 6–17 times more land than the same amount of soybean protein.

Animal protein also requires, on average, 2–3 times more water, depending on factors such as the season and annual fluctuations in rainfall.

Because of all of these factors, experts estimate that, if nothing changes, our food system will likely exceed our planet's resources by the year 2050. Switching over to a vegan diet may be one way to delay this outcome.

Types of veganism

It's important to note that vegan doesn't necessarily equal healthy.

The quality of a vegan diet depends on the foods that make it up. Thus, some vegan diets can have many health benefits, while others may not be beneficial for your health.

Here are a few subcategories of vegan diet that I've come across in my clinical practice over the last couple of years:

• **Dietary vegans.** Often used interchangeably with "plant-based eaters," this term refers to those who avoid animal products in their diet but continue to use them in other products, such as clothing and cosmetics.

• **Whole-food vegans.** These individuals favor a diet rich in whole foods, such as fruits, vegetables, whole grains, legumes, nuts, and seeds.

• **"Junk-food" vegans.** Some people rely heavily on processed vegan foods such as vegan meats, fries, frozen dinners, and desserts, including Oreo cookies and nondairy ice cream.

• **Raw-food vegans.** This group eats only foods that are raw or cooked at temperatures below 118°F (48°C).

• **Low fat raw-food vegans.** Also known as fruitarians, this subset limits high fat foods such as nuts, avocados, and coconuts, instead relying mainly on fruit. They may occasionally eat small amounts of other plants.

Whole-food vegan diets tend to offer excellent health benefits. If you're interested in trying a vegan diet, consider speaking with a healthcare professional to find the right diet for you.

Veganism and B12

Despite the many health benefits of veganism, some argue that the diet is unnatural as there aren't many plant-based sources of B12.

In the modern world, the essential vitamin is mostly found in animal products like meat and dairy. But this doesn't mean that our consumption of these is natural.

B12 is a vitamin produced by bacteria. It is created by microbes in the guts of animals and then released via their excretion. B12 is also naturally found in soil, meaning wild animals ingest it while eating plants.

Early humans likely also obtained their B12 directly from the soil while eating foraged foods. But this is no longer applicable in the modern world.

Due to the rise of intensive farming and soil degradation, the fruits and vegetables available in supermarkets do not contain B12 like produce naturally used to (especially unwashed produce). Similarly, most farmed animals don't get B12 from the soil. They are therefore supplemented, often with injections or fortified feed. This means that people who criticize veganism for its "unnatural" B12 sources are also often getting theirs indirectly via the same means.

B12 is essential for optimal human health. It is vital that vegans get their recommended daily dose of it, either via supplementation or fortified food.

What's the difference between vegan and plant-based?

Some people who adopt vegan diets for environmental or health reasons may be referred to as "plant-based." This is because they don't necessarily incorporate veganism into other aspects of their lives.

People who are "plant-based" are generally understood to avoid – or mostly avoid – animal products in their diets. They sometimes will not, however, abstain from wearing animal-based clothing or using products tested on animals. They may also support animals being used for human entertainment, such as in circuses or dolphin shows, which vegans boycott.

What's the difference between vegan and vegetarian?

While the ideas of veganism did stem from those of vegetarianism, these days they are very different lifestyles.

Broadly speaking, vegetarianism refers to people who don't eat the flesh of any dead animal, including fish and insects. They will also not eat gelatin, animal rennet, or stock made from meat. In summary, they don't eat products of animal slaughter.

They will often, however, eat eggs, dairy, honey, and some other foods made using animals. These products are acceptable for vegetarians as they aren't made directly from a dead animal.

Not all vegetarians are the same, and there will be some who choose to not eat certain animal products.

Vegetarians usually don't wear fur, and may also opt not to wear leather as well. Materials like wool and cashmere, however, will generally be accepted within the vegetarian lifestyle.

What do vegans eat?

Here are some essential foods people on a vegan diet tend to eat and avoid.

Foods that vegans eat

Avoiding animal products doesn't restrict you to eating salads and tofu alone. There's a wide variety of delicious foods you can eat on a vegan diet.

Here are a few ideas:

• Beans, peas, and lentils: such as red, brown, or green lentils; chickpeas; split peas; black-eyed peas; black beans; white beans; and kidney beans

- **Soy products:** such as fortified soy milk, soybeans, and products made from them, such as tofu, tempeh, and natto

- **Nuts:** such as peanuts, almonds, cashews, and their butters

- **Seeds:** such as sunflower seeds, sesame seeds, and their butters, as well as flaxseed, hemp seeds, and chia seeds

- **Whole grains:** such as quinoa, whole wheat, whole oats, and whole grain brown or wild rice, as well as products made from these foods, such as whole grain bread, crackers, and pasta

- **Starchy vegetables:** such as potatoes, sweet potatoes, corn, squash, beets, and turnips

- **Nonstarchy vegetables:** such as broccoli, cabbage, asparagus, radishes, and leafy greens; these may be raw, frozen, canned, dried, or pureed

• **Fruit:** such as apples, pears, bananas, berries, mango, pineapple, oranges, and tangerines; these may be purchased fresh, frozen, canned, dried, or pureed

• **Other plant-based foods:** such as algae, nutritional yeast, fortified plant milks and yogurts, and maple syrup

There's a good chance that many of the dishes you currently enjoy either already are vegan or can be made vegan with a few simple adjustments.

For instance, you can swap meat-based main dishes for meals containing beans, peas, lentils, tofu, tempeh, nuts, or seeds.

What's more, you can replace dairy products with plant milks, scrambled eggs with scrambled tofu, honey with plant-based sweeteners like molasses or maple syrup, and raw eggs with flaxseed or chia seeds.

You can also choose from the ever-growing selection of ready-made vegan products, including vegan meats, vegan cheeses, and vegan desserts.

Just keep in mind that these may be highly processed. So while they are fine to eat in moderation, they should not make up the bulk of a healthy vegan diet.

Foods that vegans avoid

Vegans avoid all foods of animal origin. These include:

• **Meat and fish**: such as beef, chicken, duck, fish, and shellfish

• **Eggs**: whole eggs and foods that contain them, such as bakery products

• **Dairy**: milk, cheese, butter, and cream, as well as foods made using these ingredients

• **Other animal-derived ingredients**: such as honey, albumin, casein, carmine, gelatin, pepsin, shellac, isinglass, and whey

Checking food labels is generally the best way to determine whether a food contains animal-derived ingredients. Many vegan foods are now also labeled as such, making it easier to recognize them when you're shopping.

Why don't vegans eat milk and eggs?

The decision not to consume animal milk (including cheese) and eggs is one of the most well-known distinguishers between vegans and vegetarians. The reason why vegans don't eat these products is because they are made from animal exploitation.

Dairy cows are farmed against their will, and it is arguable that they suffer among the worst of any animal used for food. They are forcibly impregnated each year via artificial insemination. Each time they give birth, they have their calves taken from them so that humans can drink their milk. Mother cows have been known to cry out and bellow in apparent distress for days after they're gone.

Hens used in the egg industry have been selectively bred to produce around 300 eggs a year. Naturally, it is thought they would lay just 12. Producing these eggs takes a huge toll on their bodies, and they will often suffer from osteoporosis and calcium deficiency. Many are kept in cages for their whole lives, but even those in "free-range" systems often live in cramped barns with thousands of other birds.

Further, chickens and cows used in the egg and dairy industries will end up in the slaughterhouse.

Limits of veganism

As outlined above, there are limits to how much a vegan can minimize their harm on animals.

We live in a non-vegan world. And as a result, a huge number of foods and products involve direct or indirect animal exploitation.

Some people mistakenly claim that foods like avocados and almonds aren't vegan due to the fact they rely on migratory beekeeping to be farmed.

Similarly, some argue that veganism is pointless due to the fact that many animals are killed in the gathering of crops.

It is possible to find indirect animal exploitation and death in most plant-based farming, and it would be unfeasible for vegans to avoid it all.

Vegans, therefore, are those who seek to do as much as possible to avoid animal harm in their lives.

Benefits of Combining Gluten-Free and Vegan Diets

Adopting a gluten free vegan diet can offer several health benefits. This dietary regimen, which combines the principles of a vegan lifestyle with a gluten free approach, can improve digestive health, contribute to weight management, and provide a nutrient-rich, balanced diet.

Improved Digestive Health

For individuals with celiac disease or gluten intolerance, adopting a gluten free diet can significantly improve digestive health. Gluten, a protein found in wheat, barley, and rye, can cause inflammation in the small intestine and lead to symptoms such as bloating, diarrhea, and abdominal pain. By eliminating gluten from the diet, these symptoms can be alleviated, leading to improved gut health and overall well-being.

A vegan diet, which excludes all animal products, can also contribute to better digestive health. Plant-based foods are typically high in fiber, which supports healthy gut bacteria and aids in digestion. A diet rich in fruits, vegetables, legumes, and whole grains can promote regular bowel movements and prevent constipation.

Weight Management and Heart Health

A gluten free vegan diet can also support weight management efforts. Plant-based diets are often lower in calories and saturated fats, helping to maintain a healthy weight. Additionally, many gluten-free foods are naturally lower in calories, assisting in calorie control.

Maintaining a healthy weight is crucial for heart health. Overweight and obesity are risk factors for cardiovascular diseases. By promoting weight management, a gluten free vegan diet can lower the risk of heart disease. Moreover, a plant-based diet is naturally low in cholesterol and saturated fats, further supporting cardiovascular health.

Nutrient-Rich and Balanced Diet

Despite the restrictions, a well-planned gluten free vegan diet can provide a wide array of essential nutrients. Fruits, vegetables, legumes, nuts, seeds, and gluten-free grains are all packed with vitamins, minerals, antioxidants, and dietary fiber, supporting overall health.

However, it's important to ensure that the diet is well-balanced and meets all nutritional needs. Certain nutrients, such as vitamin B12, iron, and omega-3 fatty acids, can be more challenging to obtain from a vegan diet. Likewise, individuals on a gluten-free diet should ensure that they are getting enough fiber and whole grains. Careful meal planning and a variety of gluten free vegan foods can ensure a balanced, nutrient-rich diet.

Prevention of chronic diseases

Vegan diets may be linked to a lower risk of several chronic conditions.

In fact, some research suggests that plant-based diets could be associated with a reduced risk of heart disease, type 2 diabetes, cancer, and metabolic syndrome.

Furthermore, vegan diets eliminate red meat and processed meat, both of which have been tied to an increased risk of developing certain types of cancer.

However, though some studies have found that vegan diets could be beneficial for disease prevention, more research is needed to evaluate the effects of a gluten-free, vegan diet specifically.

Nutrients and Food Sources

Vitamin B12: Fortified plant-based milks, nutritional yeast

Iron: Legumes, fortified cereals, quinoa, spinach

Omega-3 Fatty Acids: Flaxseeds, chia seeds, hemp seeds, walnuts

Overall, the gluten free vegan diet can provide numerous health benefits when followed correctly. However, it's important to consult with a healthcare professional or a dietitian to ensure that all nutritional needs are being met.

Essential Nutrients and Common Deficiencies

Vegan Diet Deficiencies

Many studies link vegetarian and vegan diets to deficiencies in key nutrients including vitamin D, magnesium, B vitamins, and iodine—all nutrients that if lacking can lead to hormonal, thyroid, and methylation impairments. Many of these nutrients are available only in animal sources, and the ones that are found in plant sources do not have the same level of bioavailability[10]. And the sources that do have decent nutrient levels also contain phytates, which end up blocking nutrient absorption.

For the most part, while vegetarian and vegan diets can both lead to major nutrient deficiencies, you typically see this less in vegetarians than in vegans because they usually still eat some type of animal product such as eggs. Either way, let's take a deeper look at the most common deficiencies and why plant-based diets don't always make the cut in this department.

DHA and EPA

Omega fatty acid deficiencies[11] in the standard vegan diet are the subject of a long-held argument. But if you are feeling better from not eating meat, is it that important to worry about not getting these omega fatty acids? A well-balanced diet with natural sources of alphalinolenic acid (ALA) and the long-chain omega-3 fatty acids DHA and EPA[11] is fundamental to maintaining a healthy ratio that prevents inflammation and promotes long-term health by protecting against health problems like autoimmune and cardiovascular disease. Additionally, your brain is composed of about 60 percent fat, so depriving your body of fat can contribute to all kinds of unpleasant brain symptoms, from brain fog and fatigue to depression and anxiety. In other words, healthy fat is essential for optimal brain health.

It is vital to consume these fatty acids because they can't be synthesized by the body, and diet is the only way to get them in. Before you argue that plant-based dieters can get these omega fats through plant-based sources such as legumes, nuts, and seeds, let's talk about how bioavailable these sources actually are.

The average American consumes a large amount of their omega-3s in the form of ALA. These are derived from plant sources. ALA is an energy source for our cells, and a small percentage of this is converted into DHA and EPA. In fact, only up to 10 percent of EPA and up to 5 percent of DHA actually end up being converted in the body. The amplest amounts are found in fatty, cold-water fish sources such as salmon, trout, cod liver, herring, mackerel, and sardines, and in shellfish such as shrimp, oysters, clams, and scallops. These sources of omega-3 are the most bioavailable to your body. Vegetarians have an estimated 30 percent deficiency in both EPA and DHA; vegans have a 50 percent deficiency in EPA and a 60 percent deficiency in DHA.

With ALA being a large source of our omega-3 consumption, and the only source for vegans, it is vital to consume DHA and EPA sources. And yes, that may mean incorporating some fish or at least algae like spirulina (which also contains bioavailable omegas) into your diet.

Vitamins A and D

Fat-soluble vitamins, in particular, are some of the worst deficiencies that we see in vegans and vegetarians. This is because these two vitamins are almost exclusively found in animal-based foods such as organ meats, eggs, dairy fats like ghee, and wild-caught seafood.

No other vitamin can hold a candle to vitamin D when it comes to importance and influence on health. Since vitamin D is fat-soluble, it acts more like a hormone than a vitamin by regulating thousands of vital pathways in your body. Besides your thyroid hormones, this vitamin is the only other thing every single cell of your body needs in order to function properly. Also known as the sunshine vitamin, vitamin D is synthesized by your body when your bare skin is exposed to sunlight. But it is impossible to get enough vitamin D from food alone, and unless you live in a very sunny place (closer to the equator) and are outside frequently without sunscreen or tons of clothing, you are probably deficient.

Since vitamin D deficiency is already a problem for most of the population, omnivores included, it is even greater for plant-based dieters. Typically, vegetarians and vegans, on average, have more vitamin D deficiencies compared to meat eaters.

Vitamin A is essential for a strong immune system, and vitamin A deficiency has been linked to autoimmune diseases19, which are on the rise in a major way. Some researchers believe this has to do with our dendritic cells, which are our alarm cells of the immune system that can send out a "red alert" to stimulate immunity or a "calm down" message that tones down excessive immune reactions that can damage the body. The "calm down" message uses vitamin A.

Plant beta-carotenes, a precursor to vitamin A, are found in sweet potatoes and carrots, but the conversion rate to the usable form of vitamin A, retinol, is very weak. In fact, research suggests that just 3 percent of beta-carotene gets converted in a healthy adult. Because of this, you can see how deficiency can be common among people who eat a vegan or vegetarian diet. You'd have to eat a rather large amount of carrots and sweet potatoes to even attempt to reach adequate levels.

Zinc

Your body has no significant way to store this important mineral, so it's important to make sure you're getting it through your diet or supplementation. Zinc's main role is to help your body increase white blood cells and fight off infection, and it also assists with the release of antibodies. Deficiency has been linked to increased instances of illness, so it's no wonder you often find zinc as a common ingredient in the cold and flu aisle of your pharmacy. It can also be especially important for pregnant women and the reduction of preterm births.

This is a very easy nutrient to get through a plant-based diet. But what we often see is that typical plant foods that contain zinc still contain phytates, which block nutrient absorption. So if intake is not monitored, zinc deficiency can still happen and often requires more zinc-containing foods to reach necessary daily intake levels.

Iron

Iron is needed to get oxygen to your cells. And if your cells are deprived of oxygen, they don't function properly and well, and not much else in your body does either. Some typical symptoms seen with low iron are fatigue and low sex drive.

There are two ways to look at iron levels in your body. One is serum iron, which measures the levels of iron currently circulating in your blood. The other is ferritin, which measures long-term iron storage in the body. The serum levels of most vegetarians and vegans are similar to those of meat eaters, but the difference is seen when it comes to ferritin levels.

While we definitely don't want ferritin levels to be too high, which is correlated with increased inflammation, we don't want them to be low either, which is a sign of iron deficiency.

There are also two different types of iron—heme and non-heme. Heme is the most bioavailable iron for your body and is found only in meat. Non-heme isn't absorbed as easily and is found in dairy, eggs, and plant foods.

Many plant foods contain iron but only the non-heme variety. Dark leafy greens, mushrooms, nuts and seeds, and legumes all contain high amounts of iron, but if you are consuming too many legumes, you'll run across problems with phytates decreasing your absorption. Additionally, iron absorption can be inhibited by other substances that are consumed such as calcium, coffee, and tea. And again, plant sources just do not have the same level of bioavailability as animal sources. All of these factors contribute to an 85 percent lower non-heme iron absorption rate in plant-based diets.

As our deficiencies continue to escalate, so does our need to supplement. For vegans and vegetarians, all of these deficiencies can be mitigated through regimented supplementation—but only if you're aware of the problems in the first place.

B12

This is potentially the biggest deficiency for all types of plant-based diets. B12 is absolutely necessary for methylation, which happens more than 1 billion times a second in your body to keep you alive and healthy. It is your DNA protection system; it controls how efficiently you detox, and every single cell of your body depends on this process. In short, if methylation is not working well, a lot can go wrong with your health.

True B12 is found only in animal products such as wild-caught fish, grass-fed beef, eggs, and dairy products. A common alternative of plant-based B12 often comes from sea vegetables like seaweed and spirulina as well as fermented soy. However, these don't contain true B12. Instead, they are B12 analogues known as cobamides, which are not as bioavailable.

For vegan and vegetarian dieters, this is one nutrient that no matter what or how much you choose to eat, you'll never truly be able to reach optimal levels without supplementation. In fact, it's estimated that 68 percent of vegetarians and 83 percent of vegans are deficient in this vital vitamin.

And that's not taking into account any possible genetic weaknesses. A mutation in your MTR/MTRR methylation gene, which regulates B12 production, can require higher intakes of B12 than normal since the body ends up using B12 faster than it can produce it.

Nutrient Deficiencies and the Gluten-Free Diet

Nutritional deficiencies can occur in individuals with celiac disease because of both low intake and poor absorption. Once the intestine has had a chance to heal, nutrient absorption improves, but intake may remain a problem. In the case of non-celiac gluten sensitivity, nutrient absorption is not compromised, but again foods consumed may be low in nutrients. Nutrient deficiencies which are common in gluten-related disorders, and their gluten-free food sources are listed in the table below.

Low intake: Very few gluten-free grain products are enriched or fortified with the vitamins and minerals that gluten-containing grain products are. Deficiencies in these vitamins and minerals can occur as a result. Some people with celiac disease also have lactose intolerance during the early stages of their treatment on a gluten-free diet, so there may be low intake of many of the nutrients provided by dairy foods (such as calcium, magnesium, and Vitamin D).

Poor absorption: When there is damage in the small intestine, the absorption of certain nutrients may be impaired. Vitamins and minerals which may be poorly absorbed include iron, calcium, folate, Vitamin B12, and all of the fat-soluble vitamins (Vitamin A, Vitamin D, Vitamin E, and Vitamin K).

Getting the Most Nutrients Out of Your Food

The nutrients in foods can vary a great deal. Here are some tips for making sure you're getting the most out of your food:

- **Eat Foods as "Whole" as Possible**: Whole, unprocessed foods have nutrients that processed foods no longer contain. Look for groceries around the perimeter of the store, because this is where most whole foods are located.

- **Cook Vegetables Lightly:** Nutrients are lost when a food is fried or boiled in water for an extended time. Lightly sauté, steam, or bake vegetables rather than frying them or boiling them in water.

- **Be Colorful:** Choose foods that are naturally bright in color. In general, each color represents a different nutrient. For example, while red tomatoes and pink watermelon have a nutrient called lycopene, orange sweet potatoes and pumpkin have a nutrient called beta-carotene. For a nutrient-rich and appetizing meal, try to include several different colors of fruits and vegetables.

CHAPTER II

TRANSITIONING TO A GLUTEN FREE VEGAN DIET

Embarking on a gluten free vegan journey can seem daunting due to some common concerns. However, with comprehensive knowledge and strategic planning, these challenges can be effectively managed.

Ensuring Adequate Protein Intake

One of the main concerns with a gluten free vegan diet is ensuring adequate protein intake. As both animal products and gluten-containing grains are excluded, alternative protein sources need to be identified.

Lentils, chickpeas, quinoa, and tofu are excellent sources of protein. Additionally, a variety of gluten free grains and seeds, such as amaranth, millet, and chia seeds, can supplement protein intake.

For a more concentrated source of protein, consider gluten free protein powders derived from peas, hemp, or brown rice.

Managing Vitamin and Mineral Levels

Another concern pertains to maintaining optimal vitamin and mineral levels, particularly Vitamin B12, iron, and calcium, which are commonly found in animal products.

To address this, incorporate foods fortified with these nutrients, like plant-based milks and breakfast cereals. Nutritional yeast is an excellent source of B12. Iron can be obtained from lentils, chickpeas, and spinach, while calcium is abundant in fortified plant milks, tofu, and certain leafy greens.

Top Tips for Starting a Gluten-Free Vegan Diet

Whether you're new to a gluten-free diet, veganism, or both, these tips will help you to get started with your new lifestyle in a healthy, sustainable way.

- Cook from scratch as often as possible so you know exactly what's going into your food.
- Focus on abundance and not restriction. There are plenty of things you can eat.
- Include plenty of healthy whole foods, and enjoy processed gluten-free alternatives in moderation.
- Get family and friends involved and organise cooking sessions with them.

- Invest in a cookbook you love or a recipe app and compile your favourite 'go-to' dishes.

How to Avoid Gluten at Home and Away

You may already be well-practised at dodging animal-products and communicating about your vegan diet, but is it so easy to dodge gluten as well?

Or, if you're new to being vegan, it could be hard to make others understand why you're going plant-based when you're already gluten-free.

Knowing how to communicate your needs, and navigate tricky situations is the key to avoiding gluten and animal products at home and away.

Explain your dietary needs to friends, family and colleagues

Being both gluten-free and vegan can be hard for some to comprehend, so try to help them understand your needs.

Most people will understand if your reasons and requirements are explained clearly, and will do their best to accommodate.

For those who find it more difficult to take on board, offer to cook with, or for, them to show them the kinds of foods you can eat, and the care you need to take over its preparation.

Cross-contamination

Educating others on your dietary needs is imperative when it comes to cross-contamination.

Having a separate area to prepare your food and using different utensils is a necessity, especially if you are coeliac.

Eating out

A lot of restaurants are well-versed in offering vegan or gluten-free options and may even offer separate menus, but it can be a challenge to combine the two.

When you eat out, be confident about asking for foods that suit your needs, look at the menu online, call the restaurant in advance or plan to go to a specific restaurant that has more choices for you.

Larger restaurants are likely to have a clear cross-contamination policy, but this is not a requirement, so be sure to ask ahead and double-check when ordering.

Know your food labels

You may be familiar with checking labels for non-vegan ingredients like milk or egg, but make sure you also check for other ingredients labelled in bold, such as wheat, barley and rye.

Wheat is a cheap, high yield product, so you'll find it in various forms used as a filler in lots of processed products.

It can crop up in some surprising places, but as gluten is in the top 14 allergens, it has to be clearly labelled in bold on food packaging.

For a product to state that it's 'gluten-free' on packaging, it has to be suitable for those with coeliac disease, which means it has to contain less than 20ppm (parts per million).

Also, remember that 'wheat free' does not necessarily mean 'gluten free'. Other grains such as barley and rye also contain gluten. Transitioning to a gluten free vegan diet can be a journey of discovering new foods, recipes, and healthier eating habits. While it may seem challenging initially, the health benefits of this lifestyle can be well worth the effort. As with any dietary change, it's always a good idea to consult with a healthcare professional or dietitian to ensure your nutritional needs are being met.

Cupboard Staples for a Gluten-Free Vegan Diet

Your diet should include plenty of fresh fruits and vegetables, and refrigerated foods like tofu and soya milk are important for protein, too.

But it can be handy to have a stock of longer-lasting staples to hand for quick meals and impromptu cooking sessions.

These are some of the most essential foods to keep in your cupboard or pantry:

Starchy carbohydrates

Naturally gluten-free options include brown rice, buckwheat, millet, teff, amaranth, sorghum and quinoa.

Potatoes and sweet potatoes with the skin on are another good source of starchy carbohydrates.

Gluten-free oats are an option, but if you have coeliac disease, check with your dietitian as some people need to exclude them.

Plant-based proteins

Many healthy plant-based proteins are naturally gluten-free, including beans, lentils, peas, peanuts, and soya foods like tempeh and tofu.

Keep a stock of these in your cupboard and you'll always have ways to make a protein-rich meal.

You may also want to keep a stock of ready-made protein options in your freezer, but keep in mind that many plant-based meat alternatives contain gluten.

Check burger, sausage and even nut roast labels thoroughly for gluten-containing ingredients and cross-contamination warnings.

There are plenty of brands these days that are both vegan and gluten-free, but these may only be available in larger supermarkets or health food stores.

Gluten-free flours

There are a range of different gluten-free flours available, and varieties made from the grains mentioned above also provide starchy carbohydrates, even when used in breads and cakes.

Almond flour, chickpea and coconut flour are also amongst the many options available, along with some specially created blends designed to mimic plain or self-raising wheat flour.

These flours can make it easy to adapt your favourite vegan recipes to be gluten-free too.

But, keep in mind that gluten-free baking often requires more moisture than traditional recipes.

It can be tricky to get the balance right, leading to dry, tough bakes.

You may prefer to find new vegan and gluten-free recipes that are tried and tested without wheat flour.

Gluten-free bread and crackers

Supermarket gluten-free breads often contain egg to help bind the ingredients together in the absence of gluten.

They also tend to use lots of other ingredients to try and mimic gluten bread, such as stabilisers, gums and additives.

Look for vegan-friendly bread made with as few ingredients as possible or try making your own.

You can make gluten-free bread using alternative flours such as chickpea and buckwheat, or buy a mix such as Orgran or Rana's Artisan Bakery.

Oat, rice or buckwheat crackers are good options for a quick, filling snack. You can make your own using alternative flour using a selection of seeds.

Making gluten-free bread involves using alternative flours and grains that are inherently gluten-free. These can include rice flour, almond flour, coconut flour, and others. A blend of these flours is typically used to mimic the texture and taste of traditional wheat bread.

To compensate for the absence of gluten, which gives bread its elasticity, other ingredients such as xanthan gum or psyllium husk might be used. These ingredients help bind the dough and create the springy texture associated with traditional bread.

Different Types of Gluten-Free Bread

There are several types of gluten-free bread available, each offering a unique taste and texture profile. Here are a few popular options:

Rice Bread

Made primarily from rice flour, this bread is light and fluffy, making it a great option for sandwiches.

Almond Bread

Almond bread, made from almond flour, has a slightly sweet, nutty flavor and is rich in protein and fiber.

Coconut Bread

Coconut bread utilizes coconut flour and has a subtly sweet flavor, making it a great choice for sweet dishes or breakfast toast.

Buckwheat Bread

Despite its name, buckwheat is completely gluten-free. Buckwheat bread has a robust, earthy flavor and is rich in nutrients.

Multigrain Bread

Multigrain gluten-free bread is made from a mix of different gluten-free flours and grains, providing a more complex flavor and added nutritional benefits.

It's important to note that while these breads are gluten-free, individuals with specific dietary needs should always check labels for additional allergens.

In the realm of gluten-free bread, there are countless options to explore, each offering their own unique taste and texture. Whether you're new to the gluten-free lifestyle or an experienced navigator, the variety of gluten-free breads available ensures that there's something to suit everyone's palate.

Gluten-free pasta

There are lots of delicious gluten-free and vegan pasta options, so there's no need to miss your favourite pasta dish.

It's best to stick to pasta found outside of the 'free-from' aisle, such as those made from chickpeas, lentils, brown rice, quinoa and mung beans, which are less processed and higher in protein.

Herbs, spices and seasonings

Both vegan and gluten-free diets have gained a bit of a reputation for being bland, but the truth is, they're anything but!

There are so many seasonings that are suitable for a gluten-free and vegan diet, so keep your cupboard well-stocked with spices and experiment with flavour combinations to keep your dishes exciting.

Be aware that some seasonings may use wheat or dairy derivatives as a bulking agent, or could be at risk of cross contamination, so always check the labels.

Soy sauce is a common choice of seasoning in a lot of vegan recipes, but this contains wheat.

Tamari is a great gluten-free alternative to soy sauce to keep on hand, or you may be able to find gluten-free soy sauce in specialist stores.

CHAPTER III

COOKING TECHNIQUES AND RECIPE MODIFICATIONS

With the rise in awareness of gluten intolerance and celiac disease, the market for gluten-free products has expanded rapidly. As a result, there are now countless gluten-free brands available, each offering a range of products to cater to different dietary needs and preferences.

Recognizing Gluten-Free Labels

When exploring gluten-free brands, it's important to understand the labeling. A product labeled as 'gluten-free' is regulated by the FDA and is required to contain less than 20 parts per million (ppm) of gluten. This is the lowest level that can be consistently detected in foods using valid scientific analytical tools.

In addition to looking for the 'gluten-free' label, also look for a certification from a recognized third-party organization like the Gluten-Free Certification Organization (GFCO). This certification is a sign that the product meets strict standards for gluten-free safety, and it is safe for those with celiac disease or gluten intolerance.

Variety of Gluten-Free Products

The range of products offered by gluten-free brands has grown significantly over the years. Now, one can find everything from gluten-free bread and pasta to snacks, desserts, and even sauces.

Besides these, there's a wide range of gluten-free grains, cereals, and flours available, making gluten-free baking a breeze. Gluten-free beverages, including beers and ciders, are also on the rise.

In the world of gluten-free brands, it's possible to find alternatives for almost every type of food product. The challenge lies in identifying the products that meet your specific dietary needs, taste preferences, and budget.

Remember, even though a product is labeled as 'gluten-free', it's still important to read the ingredient list to ensure it aligns with your overall dietary goals. For instance, some gluten-free products might be high in sugar or unhealthy fats.

Finally, it's worth noting that while packaged gluten-free products can be convenient, they should not replace a diet rich in naturally gluten-free foods like fruits, vegetables, lean proteins, and whole grains.

Important Factors When Choosing Gluten-Free Brands

When incorporating gluten-free products into your diet, it's essential to make informed choices. This involves considering several important factors such as ingredient quality and sourcing, certification and standards, and taste and texture. Let's delve into each of these aspects in detail.

Ingredient Quality and Sourcing

The quality of ingredients used in gluten-free products can greatly influence their nutritional value. Opting for brands that prioritize high-quality, natural ingredients can ensure that you're getting the most out of your gluten-free diet. This means looking for products made with whole foods, such as fruits, vegetables, and gluten-free grains.

Sourcing of ingredients is another crucial factor. Brands that are transparent about where they source their ingredients and how they are processed can provide an added level of assurance about the quality of the product. This can be particularly important for those with celiac disease or gluten intolerance, who need to avoid gluten contamination at all costs.

Certification and Standards

For those following a strict gluten-free diet, it's important to look for products that are certified gluten-free. This means the product has been tested and meets strict standards for gluten content. Brands that carry this certification will display it on their packaging.

Besides gluten-free certification, it can also be beneficial to look for brands that adhere to other quality standards, such as organic or non-GMO.

These certifications can provide additional assurance about the quality and safety of the product.

Taste and Texture

While the health aspects of gluten-free products are important, taste and texture should not be overlooked. After all, food should be enjoyed, not just consumed for health purposes.

Some gluten-free products can have a different taste or texture than their gluten-containing counterparts. Therefore, it may take some trial and error to find products that you enjoy. Whether you're looking for gluten free bread, gluten-free pasta, or gluten-free desserts, there are a variety of gluten-free brands out there that cater to different taste preferences.

Remember, choosing gluten-free brands is a personal journey and what works for one person might not work for another. Taking the time to understand these factors can help you make informed choices and find the best gluten-free brands that align with your dietary needs and preferences.

Tips for Incorporating Gluten-Free Brands into Your Diet

Transitioning to a gluten-free diet might seem challenging at first. However, with the right planning and a bit of creativity, it can be a smooth and rewarding journey. Here are some tips to incorporate gluten-free brands into your diet effectively.

Meal Planning with Gluten-Free Brands

Meal planning is a crucial step in maintaining a balanced and nourishing gluten-free diet. It involves organizing your meals and snacks for the week ahead, which can help you stay on track with your dietary goals. When planning meals, consider the variety of gluten-free foods available. From gluten-free bread and pasta to snacks and desserts, there are plenty of options to suit every taste.

Start by creating a weekly menu that includes a mix of proteins, fruits, vegetables, and gluten-free grains. Make a shopping list of ingredients you'll need, keeping an eye out for gluten-free labels when shopping. Also, consider batch cooking meals and freezing them in portions. This can save time and ensure you always have a gluten-free meal ready.

Balancing Nutrition in a Gluten-Free Diet

While focusing on gluten-free products, it's also essential to ensure a balanced diet. Some gluten-free foods might be low in certain nutrients, such as fiber and B vitamins. Make sure to include a variety of nutrient-dense foods in your diet, such as fruits, vegetables, lean proteins, and gluten-free grains.

Supplement your diet with fortified gluten-free products, which have nutrients added to them, such as iron and B vitamins. If needed, consider a multivitamin or supplement after consulting with a healthcare provider. Always remember to read labels to ensure the products are not only gluten-free but also healthy and nutritious.

Adapting Favorite Recipes to Be Gluten-Free

With a bit of creativity, most recipes can be adapted to be gluten-free. Start by swapping regular flour with gluten-free flours in your baking. There are many types available, including almond flour, coconut flour, and rice flour, each adding a unique flavor and texture to your baked goods.

Pasta dishes can be made gluten-free by using gluten-free pasta. Similarly, replace traditional breadcrumbs with gluten-free versions in recipes like meatballs or breaded chicken.

The key to successfully adapting recipes is experimentation. Don't be afraid to try different gluten-free products and see which ones work best for your favorite dishes.

Incorporating gluten-free brands into your diet doesn't have to be daunting. By planning meals, balancing nutrition, and adapting your favorite recipes, you can enjoy a diverse and satisfying gluten-free diet. Whether you're eating gluten-free due to celiac disease, gluten intolerance, or personal preference, these strategies can help you embrace a healthier you.

CHAPTER IV

EXPLORING GLUTEN-FREE BAKING

Many people are now turning towards gluten-free baking as a healthier option to traditional baking. This shift is not only beneficial for those with gluten intolerance or celiac disease, but also for anyone seeking to improve their overall health.

Health Benefits of Gluten-Free Baking

One of the main health benefits of gluten-free baking is that it can aid in digestion. Gluten, a protein found in wheat, barley, and rye, can cause digestive issues in some individuals, particularly those with celiac disease or gluten intolerance. By eliminating gluten from your baking, you can reduce these symptoms and improve your gut health.

Moreover, gluten-free baking often involves using nutrient-rich, alternative flour sources such as almond flour, coconut flour, or gluten-free flours made from grains like quinoa and buckwheat. These alternatives offer a range of vitamins, minerals, and fiber that can contribute to a well-rounded diet.

Lastly, gluten-free baking can also contribute to weight management. Many gluten-free ingredients are lower in carbohydrates than their gluten-containing counterparts, which could help those looking to manage their weight or blood sugar levels.

Flavor and Texture: The Gluten-Free Difference

Not only does gluten-free baking offer health advantages, but it also introduces a unique flavor and texture profile to baked goods. Alternative flours bring their own distinct tastes that can elevate the flavor of your baking, creating a new taste experience.

The texture of gluten-free baked goods can vary greatly depending on the ingredients used. For example, almond flour can lend a moist, dense texture to cakes and muffins, while coconut flour can result in a fluffier, more delicate crumb.

The key to mastering gluten-free baking lies in understanding how different ingredients work together to mimic the structure and texture that gluten usually provides. With the right mix of ingredients, it's possible to create gluten-free baked goods that are just as delicious, if not more so, than traditional baked goods.

In the end, gluten-free baking is not just about eliminating gluten, but about exploring a whole new world of flavors, textures, and ingredients. Whether you're gluten intolerant or simply looking to diversify your diet, gluten-free baking can be a delicious and nutritious addition to your culinary repertoire.

Essential Gluten-Free Baking Directions

Baking in a gluten-free way requires a shift from traditional ingredients to alternatives that deliver similar results. In gluten-free baking, three types of ingredients play a critical role: gluten-free flours, binding agents, and sweeteners and flavor enhancers.

Gluten-Free Flours

Gluten-free flours form the foundation of gluten-free baking. These flours are derived from a variety of sources, including grains, nuts, seeds, and legumes. Some popular choices include almond flour, coconut flour, rice flour, and buckwheat flour. Each flour brings a distinct flavor and texture to the baked goods, so it's often beneficial to combine several types to achieve the desired result.

Sources of Gluten-Free Flour

Almond Flour: Almonds

Coconut Flour: Coconut Meat

Rice Flour: Rice

Buckwheat Flour: Buckwheat Seeds

Binding Agents in Gluten-Free Baking

In the absence of gluten, a binding agent is needed to provide structure and prevent the baked goods from falling apart. These agents mimic the role of gluten, providing elasticity and moisture. Some commonly used binding agents in gluten-free baking include xanthan gum and guar gum. Eggs are also a natural binding agent and can contribute to the texture and rise of the baked goods.

Role of Binding Agent

Xanthan Gum Mimics Gluten, Provides Elasticity

Guar Gum Improves Texture, Provides Moisture

Eggs Acts as Natural Binder, Contributes to Rise

Sweeteners and Flavor Enhancers

Sweeteners and flavor enhancers are crucial in gluten-free baking. They enhance the taste and texture of the baked goods, making them more palatable. Commonly used sweeteners include honey, maple syrup, and coconut sugar. Flavor enhancers can be anything from vanilla extract to spices like cinnamon and nutmeg. The choice of sweeteners and flavor enhancers can greatly impact the overall taste of the baked goods, so it's important to choose them wisely.

Sweetener/Flavor Enhancer Role

Honey: Natural Sweetener

Maple Syrup: Natural Sweetener

Vanilla Extract: Flavor Enhancer

Cinnamon: Flavor Enhancer

Understanding these ingredients and their roles can greatly enhance your gluten-free baking experience. Remember, it may take some time to get used to these ingredients and to learn how to combine them effectively. Don't be afraid to experiment and adjust the recipes to your liking.

Tips for Successful Gluten-Free Baking

Mastering the art of gluten-free baking can be a rewarding adventure. However, it does require a few adjustments to traditional baking techniques. Let's explore some helpful tips that will assist you in creating delicious and nutritious gluten-free baked goods.

Adjusting Traditional Baking Techniques

When it comes to gluten-free baking, a one-size-fits-all approach doesn't always work. Conventional recipes usually rely on gluten, a protein in wheat, to provide structure and elasticity. Since gluten-free flours lack this protein, you may need to modify your baking techniques.

For instance, over mixing dough in traditional baking can result in tough and chewy baked goods due to the development of gluten. However, in gluten-free baking, you can't overdevelop gluten, so don't be afraid to mix your batter thoroughly to ensure all ingredients are well incorporated.

Additionally, you may need to bake gluten-free goods at a lower temperature for a longer time. This can help to avoid the common issue of the crust browning too quickly before the inside is fully cooked.

Ensuring Moisture and Flavor Balance

Gluten-free flours typically absorb more moisture than their gluten-containing counterparts, which can lead to dry and crumbly baked goods. To counteract this, consider adding extra liquid to your recipes or using moist ingredients like applesauce, mashed bananas, or yogurt.

Flavor is another important aspect to consider. Some gluten-free flours have distinct tastes that can alter the flavor of your baked goods. It can be beneficial to use a blend of different flours or to add extra spices, extracts, or flavor enhancers to balance out the taste.

Troubleshooting Common Gluten-Free Baking Issues

Even with careful preparation, you might encounter some common issues in gluten-free baking. Here are a few troubleshooting tips:

1. **Dry and crumbly texture**: Try adding more liquid, using a blend of gluten-free flours, or incorporating a binding agent like xanthan gum to provide structure and moisture.

2. **Gummy or dense texture:** This can occur if too much xanthan gum or other binding agent is used. Try reducing the amount in your recipe.

3. **Baked goods not rising**: Gluten-free baked goods often need help to rise. Consider using a combination of baking powder, baking soda, and an acid (like vinegar or lemon juice) to help your baked goods puff up.

Remember, successful gluten-free baking often involves some trial and error. Don't be discouraged if your first few attempts don't turn out perfectly. With practice and patience, you can create delicious and healthy gluten-free baked goods that rival their gluten-filled counterparts.

Delicious Gluten-Free Baking Recipes

Pivoting to a gluten-free diet doesn't mean giving up on the joy of baking. There is an array of gluten-free baking recipes that offer appetizing alternatives to traditional baked goods. This section provides a glimpse into the variety of gluten-free bread, cakes, cookies, and savory bakes that can be easily made at home.

Gluten-Free Bread Varieties

Making gluten-free bread at home can be a satisfying experience. It involves combining gluten-free flours, such as rice flour, almond flour, or potato starch, with binding agents like xanthan gum or psyllium husk to create a dough that rises well and retains its structure post baking. Some popular gluten-free bread varieties include:

1. **Gluten-Free Multigrain Bread:** This wholesome bread combines a mix of gluten-free grains and seeds for added texture and nutritional value.

2. **Gluten-Free Sourdough Bread:** Made with a gluten-free sourdough starter, this bread has a distinctive tangy flavor that sourdough lovers will appreciate.

3. **Gluten-Free Banana Bread:** A sweet, moist bread that's perfect for breakfast or a snack. It's a great way to use up overripe bananas.

Gluten-Free Cakes and Cookies

Gluten-free cakes and cookies can be just as delightful as their gluten-filled counterparts. Here are a few favorites:

1. **Gluten-Free Chocolate Cake**: A rich, moist chocolate cake that uses gluten-free flour for a delicious dessert that everyone can enjoy.

2. **Gluten-Free Vanilla Cupcakes**: Light and fluffy cupcakes made with a simple gluten-free flour blend and pure vanilla extract.

3. **Gluten-Free Chocolate Chip Cookies**: These cookies use almond flour and gluten-free oats for a perfect balance of crispy edges and a soft middle.

Gluten-Free Savory Bakes

From pies to quiches and pastries, there are numerous gluten-free savory bakes to explore:

1. **Gluten-Free Pizza Crust**: A pizza crust made from a blend of gluten-free flours and yeast for a dough that's easy to work with and bakes up crispy and delicious.

2. **Gluten-Free Quiche**: A fluffy, custard-like filling baked in a gluten-free pie crust. Add your favorite vegetables, cheese, and meats for a customizable meal.

3. **Gluten-Free Vegetable Tart:** A savory tart filled with seasonal vegetables and a creamy custard, encased in a gluten-free pastry crust.

These gluten-free baking recipes showcase the versatility and deliciousness of gluten-free baking. Whether you're new to the world of gluten-free baking or an experienced baker looking for new recipes to try, there's plenty to choose from. Enjoy exploring these options and creating your own delicious gluten-free baked goods.

Nutritional Considerations in Gluten-Free Baking

While gluten-free baking offers several health benefits, it's crucial to consider the nutritional aspects. Gluten-free flours are often made from grains like rice, corn, and quinoa, or from nuts and legumes. These alternatives can provide a range of nutrients, but their nutritional profiles differ from traditional wheat flour.

For instance, gluten-free flours may have lower levels of certain nutrients, such as fiber and B vitamins. However, they can also provide other benefits, like increased protein content in the case of legume-based flours. To ensure a balanced diet, consider incorporating a variety of gluten-free grains and gluten-free flours into your baking.

CHAPTER V

NOURISHING GLUTEN-FREE

VEGAN RECIPES FOR EVERYDAY

NOURISHING GLUTEN-FREE VEGAN BREAKFAST IDEAS

Apricot & hazelnut muesli

INGREDIENTS

- 250g porridge oats

- 75g blanched hazelnuts, halved

- 75g pumpkin seeds

- 1 ½ tsp ground cinnamon

- 75g sulphur-free dried apricots, chopped

- 20g apple fruit crisps, or dried apple

- 600ml fortified oat milk

• 240g blueberries

INSTRUCTIONS

• STEP 1

Toast the porridge oats in a frying pan over a gentle heat, stirring frequently. Turn off the heat and stir in the nuts, seeds and cinnamon until fully combined.

• STEP 2

Tip into a large bowl, stirring to help it cool, then add the fruit, breaking the apple crisps into smaller pieces. Toss to combine.

• STEP 3

 Serve the rest in a bowl with 100ml milk and 40g berries in each.

Millet porridge with almond milk & berry compote

INGREDIENTS

- 340g millet

- 1 litre unsweetened fortified almond milk, plus extra to serve

- few mint leaves, to serve

For the compote

- 90g pitted dates, finely chopped

- 500g frozen mixed fruit (ours was a mixed bag of berries, cherries, currants and strawberries)

- 1 cinnamon stick

INSTRUCTIONS

• STEP 1

For the compote, put the dates in a pan with 150ml water, bring to the boil and stir well so they break down. Tip in the frozen fruit and cinnamon stick and cook over a medium heat, stirring every now and then for a couple of minutes. Don't worry about fully thawing larger fruits, as they will defrost in the residual heat and retain their shape in the compote (if you have large strawberries in the mix, you can halve these as they soften). Leave to cool. Will then keep chilled for up to four days.

• STEP 2

Rinse the millet in a sieve, then tip into a deep, heavy-based saucepan and pour in the almond milk and 350ml water. Put over a low heat and once bubbling, leave to simmer for 10-12 mins, stirring frequently until the millet grains are tender, but nutty.

• STEP 3

Serve the porridge with the compote. Add a little extra almond milk to serve with a few mint leaves scattered over.

Oat & chia porridge

INGREDIENTS

• 150g porridge oats

• 50g milled seeds with flax and chia

• 400ml fortified oat milk

• 200g coconut yogurt

• 40g flaked almonds,toasted

• 2 pink grapefruit, segmented and chopped (4 portions)

INSTRUCTIONS

• STEP 1

Soak the oats and seeds in 800ml water overnight. Toast your flaked almonds in a dry frying pan over a medium heat until golden brown on each side, about 2-3mins. Set aside in an airtight container.

• STEP 2

Tip into a pan with 200ml oat milk and heat, stirring, until bubbling and thick. Divide into bowls, along with 50ml oat milk each and topping with a quarter portion each of the yogurt, almonds and grapefruit.

Tofu scramble

INGREDIENTS

* 1 tbsp olive oil

* 1 small onion, finely sliced

* 1 large garlic clove, crushed

* ½ tsp turmeric

* 1 tsp ground cumin

* ½ tsp sweet smoked paprika

* 280g extra firm tofu

* 100g cherry tomatoes, halved

* ½ small bunch parsley, chopped

* rye bread, to serve, (optional)

INSTRUCTIONS

* STEP 1

Heat the oil in a frying pan over a medium heat and gently fry the onion for 8 -10 mins or until golden brown and sticky. Stir in the garlic, turmeric, cumin and paprika and cook for 1 min.

• STEP 2

Roughly mash the tofu in a bowl using a fork, keeping some pieces chunky. Add to the pan and fry for 3 mins. Raise the heat, then tip in the tomatoes, cooking for 5 mins more or until they begin to soften. Fold the parsley through the mixture. Serve on its own or with toasted rye bread (not gluten-free), if you like.

Ultimate Seville orange marmalade

INGREDIENTS

• 1.3kg Seville orange

- 2 lemons, juice only

- 2.6kg preserving or granulated sugar

INSTRUCTIONS

- STEP 1

Put the whole oranges and lemon juice in a large preserving pan and cover with 2 litres/4 pints water - if it does not cover the fruit, use a smaller pan. If necessary weight the oranges with a heat-proof plate to keep them submerged. Bring to the boil, cover and simmer very gently for around 2 hours, or until the peel can be easily pierced with a fork.

- STEP 2

Warm half the sugar in a very low oven. Pour off the cooking water from the oranges into a jug and tip the oranges into a bowl. Return cooking liquid to the pan. Allow oranges to cool until they are easy to handle, then cut in half. Scoop out all the pips and pith and add to the reserved orange liquid in the pan. Bring to the boil for 6 minutes, then strain this liquid through a sieve into a bowl and press the pulp through with a wooden spoon - it is high in pectin so gives marmalade a good set.

• STEP 3

Pour half this liquid into a preserving pan. Cut the peel, with a sharp knife, into fine shreds. Add half the peel to the liquid in the preserving pan with the warm sugar. Stir over a low heat until all the sugar has dissolved, for about 10 minutes, then bring to the boil and bubble rapidly for 15- 25 minutes until setting point is reached.

• STEP 4

Take pan off the heat and skim any scum from the surface. (To dissolve any excess scum, drop a small knob of butter on to the surface, and gently stir.) Leave the marmalade to stand in the pan for 20 minutes to cool a little and allow the peel to settle; then pot in sterilised jars, seal and label. Repeat from step 3 for second batch, warming the other half of the sugar first.

Instant berry banana slush

INGREDIENTS

• 2 ripe bananas

• 200g frozen berry mix (blackberries, raspberries and currants)

INSTRUCTIONS

• STEP 1

Slice the bananas into a bowl and add the frozen berry mix. Blitz with a stick blender to make a slushy ice and serve straight away in two glasses with spoons.

Tofu brekkie pancakes

INGREDIENTS

• 50g Brazil nuts

• 3 sliced bananas

• 240g raspberries

• maple syrup or honey, to serve

For the batter

• 349g pack firm silken tofu

• 2 tsp vanilla extract

* 2 tsp lemon juice

* 400ml unsweetened almond milk

* 1 tbsp vegetable oil, plus 1-2 tbsp extra for frying

* 250g buckwheat flour

* 4 tbsp light muscovado sugar

* 1 ½ tsp ground mixed spice

* 1 tbsp gluten-free baking powder

INSTRUCTIONS

* STEP 1

Heat oven to 180C/160C fan/gas 4. Scatter the nuts over a baking tray and cook for 5 mins until toasty and golden. Leave to cool, then chop. Turn the oven down low if you want to keep the whole batch of pancakes warm, although I think they are best enjoyed straight from the pan.

• STEP 2

Put the tofu, vanilla, lemon juice and 200ml of the milk into a deep jug or bowl. Using a stick blender, blend together until liquid, then keep going until it turns thick and smooth, like yogurt. Stir in the oil and the rest of the milk to loosen the mixture.

• STEP 3

Put the dry ingredients and 1 tsp salt in a large bowl and whisk to combine and aerate. If there are any lumps in the sugar, squish them with your fingers. Make a well in the centre, pour in the tofu mix and bring together to make a thick batter.

• STEP 4

Heat a large (ideally non-stick) frying pan and swirl around 1 tsp oil. For golden pancakes that don't stick, the pan and oil should be hot enough to get an enthusiastic sizzle on contact with the batter, but not so hot that it scorches it. Test a drop.

• STEP 5

Using a ladle or large serving spoon, drop in 3 spoonfuls of batter, easing it out gently in the pan to make pancakes that are about 12cm across. Cook for 2 mins on the first side or until bubbles pop over most of the surface. Loosen with a palette knife, then flip over the pancakes and cook for 1 min more or until puffed up and firm. Transfer to the oven to keep warm, if you need to, but don't stack the pancakes too closely. Cook the rest of the batter, using a little more oil each time. Serve warm with sliced banana, berries, toasted nuts and a good drizzle of maple syrup or honey.

Coconut Blueberry Smoothie

INGREDIENTS

• ¼ cup light coconut milk

• ¼ cup orange juice

• 2 tablespoons coconut cream

• 1 cup frozen blueberries

• 1 tablespoon maple syrup (Optional)

INSTRUCTIONS

1. Add coconut milk, orange juice, coconut cream, blueberries and maple syrup (if using) to a blender. Blend until smooth.

Chocolate Banana Oatmeal

INGREDIENTS

• 1 cup water

• Pinch of salt

• ½ cup old-fashioned rolled oats

• ½ small banana, sliced

• 1 tablespoon chocolate-hazelnut spread

• Pinch of flaky sea salt

INSTRUCTIONS

1. Bring water and a pinch of regular salt to a boil in a small saucepan. Stir in oats, reduce heat to medium and cook, stirring occasionally, until most of the liquid is absorbed, about 5 minutes. Remove

from heat, cover and let stand 2 to 3 minutes. Top with banana, chocolate spread and flaky salt.

Tips

Overnight oats variation

Combine 1/2 cup old-fashioned rolled oats with 1/2 cup water and a pinch of salt in a jar or bowl or jar. Cover and refrigerate overnight. In the morning, add toppings. Eat cold or heat up. Makes about 1 cup.

Steel-cut oats variation

Bring 1 cup water and a pinch of salt to a boil in a small saucepan. Add 1/3 cup steel-cut oats, reduce heat to a bare simmer, cover and cook, stirring occasionally, until most of the liquid is absorbed, 15 to 20 minutes. Remove from heat and let stand, covered, 2 to 3 minutes. Add toppings. Makes about 1 cup.

People with celiac disease or gluten-sensitivity should use oats that are labeled "gluten-free," as oats are often cross-contaminated with wheat and barley.

Strawberry-Pineapple Smoothie

INGREDIENTS

• 1 cup frozen strawberries

• 1 cup chopped fresh pineapple

• ¾ cup chilled unsweetened almond milk, plus more if needed

• 1 tablespoon almond butter

INSTRUCTIONS

1. Combine strawberries, pineapple, almond milk and almond butter in a blender. Process until

smooth, adding more almond milk, if needed, for desired consistency. Serve immediately.

Carrot-Apple Smoothie

INGREDIENTS

• 2 large carrots, sliced (about 1 1/2 cups)

• 1 medium-ripe banana

• 1 large Honeycrisp apple, cored and quartered

• 1 cup light coconut milk

• 2 tablespoons fresh lemon juice

• 2 teaspoons minced fresh ginger

• 2 teaspoons minced fresh turmeric or 1 teaspoon ground turmeric

• ½ cup ice cubes

INSTRUCTIONS

1. Combine carrots, banana, apple, coconut milk, lemon juice, ginger and turmeric in a blender. Process until smooth, about 45 seconds. Add ice cubes and process until smooth, about 30 seconds. Serve immediately.

Quick-Cooking Oats

INGREDIENTS

• 1 cup water or low-fat milk

• Pinch of salt

• ½ cup quick-cooking oats (see Tip)

• 1 ounce low-fat milk for serving

• 1 to 2 teaspoons honey, cane sugar or brown sugar for serving

• Pinch of cinnamon

INSTRUCTIONS

1. Stovetop: Combine water (or milk) and salt in a small saucepan. Bring to a boil. Stir in oats and reduce heat to medium; cook for 1 minute. Remove from heat, cover and let stand for 2 to 3 minutes.

2. Microwave: Combine water (or milk), salt and oats in a 2-cup microwave-safe bowl. Microwave on High for 1 1/2 to 2 minutes. Stir before serving.

3. Serve with your favorite toppings, such as milk, sweetener, cinnamon, dried fruits and nuts.

Strawberry-Mango-Banana Smoothie

INGREDIENTS

• ½ cup frozen strawberries

• ½ cup chopped ripe mango

• ½ medium ripe banana (frozen, if desired)

• ½ cup unsweetened refrigerated coconut milk beverage (such as So Delicious), plus more if needed

• 1 tablespoon cashew butter

• 1 tablespoon ground chia seeds

INSTRUCTIONS

1. Combine strawberries, mango, banana, coconut milk, cashew butter and chia seeds in a blender. Process until smooth, adding more coconut milk, if needed, for desired consistency. Serve immediately.

Berry-Banana Cauliflower Smoothie

INGREDIENTS

• 1 cup frozen riced cauliflower

• ½ cup frozen mixed berries

• 1 cup sliced frozen banana

• 2 cups unsweetened plain almond milk

• 2 teaspoons maple syrup

INSTRUCTIONS

1. Place cauliflower, berries, banana, almond milk and maple syrup in a blender; blend until smooth, 3 to 4 minutes.

NOURISHING GLUTEN-FREE VEGAN LUNCH RECIPES

Brussels Sprouts Salad with Crunchy Chickpeas

INGREDIENTS

• 1 (9 to 10 ounce) package shredded or shaved Brussels sprouts

• 4 cups chopped kale

• 1/2 cup Tahini Sauce with Lemon & Garlic

• 1 cup roasted chickpea snacks with sea salt

• 1 medium avocado, pitted and quartered

INSTRUCTIONS

1. Divide Brussels sprouts and kale among 4 single-serving lidded containers (you'll have about 3 1/2 cups of greens in each container). Seal and refrigerate for up to 4 days.

2. Transfer 2 tablespoons tahini sauce into each of 4 small lidded containers; refrigerate for up to 4 days.

3. Just before serving each salad, drizzle with 1 portion of tahini sauce and toss well to coat. Top with 1/4 cup roasted chickpeas and 1/4 avocado.

Vegan Grain Bowl

INGREDIENTS

• 1 medium sweet potato, peeled if desired, cut into 1-inch chunks

• 3 tablespoons extra-virgin olive oil, divided

- ½ teaspoon salt, divided

- ½ teaspoon ground pepper, divided

- 2 tablespoons tahini

- 2 tablespoons water

- 1 tablespoon lemon juice

- 1 small clove garlic, minced

- 2 cups cooked quinoa

- 1 15-ounce can chickpeas, rinsed

- 1 firm ripe avocado, diced

- ¼ cup chopped fresh cilantro or parsley

INSTRUCTIONS

1. Preheat oven to 425 degrees F.

2. Toss sweet potato with 1 tablespoon oil and 1/4 teaspoon each salt and pepper in a medium bowl. Transfer to a rimmed baking sheet. Roast, stirring once, until tender, 15 to 18 minutes.

3. Meanwhile, whisk the remaining 2 tablespoons oil, tahini, water, lemon juice, garlic and the remaining 1/4 teaspoon each salt and pepper in a small bowl.

4. To serve, divide quinoa among 4 bowls. Top with equal amounts of sweet potato, chickpeas and avocado. Drizzle with the tahini sauce. Sprinkle with parsley (or cilantro).

Stuffed Sweet Potato with Hummus Dressing

INGREDIENTS

• 1 large sweet potato, scrubbed

• ¾ cup chopped kale

• 1 cup canned black beans, rinsed

• ¼ cup hummus

• 2 tablespoons water

INSTRUCTIONS

1. Prick sweet potato all over with a fork. Microwave on High until cooked through, 7 to 10 minutes.

2. Meanwhile, wash kale and drain, allowing water to cling to the leaves. Place in a medium saucepan; cover and cook over medium-high heat, stirring once or twice, until wilted. Add beans; add a tablespoon or two of water if the pot is dry. Continue cooking, uncovered, stirring occasionally, until the mixture is steaming hot, 1 to 2 minutes.

3. Split the sweet potato open and top with the kale and bean mixture. Combine hummus and 2 tablespoons water in a small dish. Add additional water as needed to reach desired consistency. Drizzle the hummus dressing over the stuffed sweet potato.

Chopped Salad with Sriracha Tofu & Peanut Dressing

INGREDIENTS

• 1 (10 ounce) package kale, Brussels sprout, broccoli and cabbage salad mix

• 1 (12 ounce) package frozen shelled edamame, thawed

• 2 (7 ounce) packages Sriracha-flavored baked tofu, cubed

• 1/2 cup spicy peanut vinaigrette

INSTRUCTIONS

1. Divide salad mix among 4 single-serving containers with lids. Top each with 1/2 cup edamame and one-fourth of the tofu.

2. Transfer 2 tablespoons vinaigrette into each of 4 small lidded containers and refrigerate for up to 4 days.

3. Seal the salad containers and refrigerate for up to 4 days. Dress with vinaigrette up to 1 day before serving.

Tips

To make ahead: Refrigerate for up to 4 days.

Roasted Veggie & Tofu Brown Rice Bowl

INGREDIENTS

• ½ cup cooked brown rice

• 1 cup roasted vegetables

• 1 cup roasted tofu

• 2 tablespoons sliced scallions

• 2 tablespoons chopped fresh cilantro

• 2 tablespoons Creamy Vegan Cashew Sauce

INSTRUCTIONS

1. Arrange rice, veggies and tofu in a bowl or 4-cup sealable container. Sprinkle with scallions and cilantro. When ready to serve, top with cashew sauce.

Quinoa, Avocado & Chickpea Salad over Mixed Greens

INGREDIENTS

- ⅔ cup water

- ⅓ cup quinoa

- ¼ teaspoon kosher salt or other coarse salt

- 1 clove garlic, crushed and peeled

- 2 teaspoons grated lemon zest

- 3 tablespoons lemon juice

- 3 tablespoons olive oil

- ¼ teaspoon ground pepper

- 1 cup rinsed no-salt-added canned chickpeas

• 1 medium carrot, shredded (1/2 cup)

• ½ avocado, diced

• 1 (5 ounce) package prewashed mixed greens, such as spring mix or baby kale-spinach blend (8 cups packed)

INSTRUCTIONS

1. Bring water to a boil in a small saucepan. Stir in quinoa. Reduce heat to low, cover, and simmer until all the liquid is absorbed, about 15 minutes. Use a fork to fluff and separate the grains; let cool for 5 minutes.

2. Meanwhile, sprinkle salt over garlic on a cutting board. Mash the garlic with the side of a spoon until a paste forms. Scrape into a medium bowl. Whisk in lemon zest, lemon juice, oil, and pepper. Transfer 3 Tbsp. of the dressing to a small bowl and set aside.

3. Add chickpeas, carrot, and avocado to the bowl with the remaining dressing; gently toss to combine. Let stand for 5 minutes to allow flavors to blend. Add the quinoa and gently toss to coat.

4. Place greens in a large bowl and toss with the reserved 3 Tbsp. dressing. Divide the greens between 2 plates and top with the quinoa mixture.

Tips

To make ahead: Prepare quinoa (Step 1) and refrigerate for up to 2 days.

Edamame & Veggie Rice Bowl

INGREDIENTS

• ½ cup cooked brown rice

• 1 cup roasted vegetables

• ¼ cup edamame

• ¼ avocado, diced

• 2 tablespoons sliced scallions

• 2 tablespoons chopped fresh cilantro

• 2 tablespoons Citrus-Lime Vinaigrette

INSTRUCTIONS

1. Arrange rice, veggies, edamame and avocado in a 4-cup sealable container or bowl. Top with scallions and cilantro. Drizzle with vinaigrette just before serving.

Roasted Veggie Mason Jar Salad

INGREDIENTS

• 2 tablespoons Creamy Vegan Cashew Sauce

- 1 cup roasted tofu

- 1 tablespoon pumpkin seeds

- 1 cup roasted vegetables

- 2 cups mixed greens

INSTRUCTIONS

1. Layer into a 4-cup jar, in this order: sauce, tofu, pumpkin seeds, veggies and greens. Close tightly and refrigerate for up to 5 days.

Grain Bowl with Chickpeas & Cauliflower

INGREDIENTS

- 1 cup small cauliflower florets

- 1 teaspoon extra-virgin olive oil

- ½ teaspoon ground cumin

- ¼ teaspoon salt, divided

- 3 tablespoons hot tap water

- 2 tablespoons tahini

- 1 tablespoon lemon juice

- 1 clove garlic, minced

- 1 teaspoon za'atar

- 1 ½ cups baby kale

- ½ cup cooked quinoa

- ½ cup canned chickpeas, rinsed

INSTRUCTIONS

1. Preheat oven to 425 degrees F.

2. Toss cauliflower with oil, cumin and 1/8 teaspoon salt in a medium bowl. Transfer to a small baking

dish; roast until the cauliflower is tender, 12 to 15 minutes.

3. Meanwhile, whisk water, tahini, lemon juice, garlic, za'atar and the remaining 1/8 teaspoon salt in a small bowl.

4. Place kale in the bottom of a shallow serving bowl. Top with cauliflower, quinoa and chickpeas; drizzle with 2 tablespoons of the dressing (save the rest for another use).

Curried Sweet Potato & Peanut Soup

INGREDIENTS

• 2 tablespoons canola oil

• 1 ½ cups diced yellow onion

• 1 tablespoon minced garlic

- 1 tablespoon minced fresh ginger

- 4 teaspoons red curry paste (see Tip)

- 1 serrano chile, ribs and seeds removed, minced

- 1 pound sweet potatoes, peeled and cubed (1/2-inch pieces)

- 3 cups water

- 1 cup "lite" coconut milk

- ¾ cup unsalted dry-roasted peanuts

- 1 (15 ounce) can white beans, rinsed

- ¾ teaspoon salt

- ¼ teaspoon ground pepper

- ¼ cup chopped fresh cilantro

- 2 tablespoons lime juice

• ¼ cup unsalted roasted pumpkin seeds

• Lime wedges

INSTRUCTIONS

1. Heat oil in a large pot over medium-high heat. Add onion and cook, stirring often, until softened and translucent, about 4 minutes.

2. Stir in garlic, ginger, curry paste, and serrano; cook, stirring, for 1 minute. Stir in sweet potatoes and water; bring to a boil. Reduce heat to medium-low and simmer, partially covered, until the sweet potatoes are soft, 10 to 12 minutes.

3. Transfer half of the soup to a blender, along with coconut milk and peanuts; puree. (Use caution when pureeing hot liquids.) Return to the pot with the remaining soup. Stir in beans, salt, and pepper; heat through. Remove from the heat. Stir in cilantro

and lime juice. Serve with pumpkin seeds and lime wedges.

Tips

Tip: You can find red curry paste in the Asian section of many grocery stores, packaged in a small glass jar.

Crunchy Mexican Salad with Spicy Cilantro Vinaigrette

INGREDIENTS

• 2 cups Veggie Crunch Salad

• ½ cup rinsed canned low-sodium black beans

• ½ cup diced red bell pepper

• 2 tablespoons fresh cilantro leaves

• 2 tablespoons roasted, salted pumpkin seeds

• 2 tablespoons Cilantro-Lime Vinaigrette

INSTRUCTIONS

1. Pack salad, beans, bell pepper, cilantro and pumpkin seeds in an airtight storage container or large mason jar. Pack vinaigrette separately in a small jar. Just before eating, add the vinaigrette to the salad and toss.

Vegan Burrito Bowls with Cauliflower Rice

INGREDIENTS

• 1 recipe Tofu Crumbles

• 1 (12 ounce) package frozen riced cauliflower

• 4 teaspoons olive oil

• 1 teaspoon no-salt-added taco seasoning

• 1 cup thinly sliced red cabbage

• 1 cup diced avocado

• ½ cup pico de gallo or salsa

• ¼ cup chopped fresh cilantro

INSTRUCTIONS

1. Prepare Tofu Crumbles as directed.

2. While the Tofu Crumbles cook, prepare riced cauliflower according to package **Directions**. Toss with oil and taco seasoning.

3. Divide the cauliflower among 4 single-serving containers with lids. Top each with 1/2 cup Tofu Crumbles, 1/4 cup each cabbage and avocado, 2 tablespoons pico de gallo (or salsa) and 1 tablespoon

cilantro. Seal the containers and refrigerate until ready to eat.

Tofu & Roasted Vegetable Grain Bowl with Pumpkin Seeds

INGREDIENTS

• 8 ounces extra-firm tofu, cut into 1-inch cubes

• 5 tablespoons plus 1 teaspoon extra-virgin olive oil, divided

• 1 tablespoon reduced-sodium tamari or soy sauce (see Tip)

• ½ teaspoon chili powder

• 1 medium red bell pepper, cut into 1/2-inch strips

• ½ medium red onion, cut into 1/2-inch wedges

• ½ avocado

• ⅓ cup water

• ¼ cup packed cilantro leaves, plus more for garnish

• 2 tablespoons lime juice

• ½ teaspoon ground coriander

• ¼ teaspoon salt

• 1 cup cooked brown rice

• ½ cup chopped romaine lettuce

• 6 cherry tomatoes, halved

• 2 tablespoons toasted pumpkin seeds

INSTRUCTIONS

1. Preheat oven to 425 degrees F. Line a rimmed baking sheet with parchment paper.

2. Toss tofu, 1 tablespoon oil, tamari (or soy sauce) and chili powder in a medium bowl. Place on one side of the prepared baking sheet. Add pepper, onion and 1 teaspoon oil to the bowl; stir to coat. Place the vegetables on the other side of the baking sheet. Roast until the vegetables are tender and the tofu is sizzling, about 20 minutes.

3. Meanwhile, combine the remaining 4 tablespoons oil, avocado, water, cilantro, lime juice, coriander and salt in a blender jar or mini food processor. Process until smooth, scraping the sides down as necessary.

4. Place 1/2 cup rice in each of 2 shallow serving bowls. Top with the tofu, roasted vegetables, lettuce and tomatoes. Spoon 4 tablespoons dressing over each bowl and sprinkle with pumpkin seeds.

Weight-Loss Cabbage Soup

INGREDIENTS

- 2 tablespoons extra-virgin olive oil

- 1 medium onion, chopped

- 2 medium carrots, chopped

- 2 stalks celery, chopped

- 1 medium red bell pepper, chopped

- 2 cloves garlic, minced

- 1 ½ teaspoons Italian seasoning

- ½ teaspoon ground pepper

- ¼ teaspoon salt

- 8 cups low-sodium vegetable broth

• 1 medium head green cabbage, halved and sliced

• 1 large tomato, chopped

• 2 teaspoons white-wine vinegar

INSTRUCTIONS

1. Heat oil in a large pot over medium heat. Add onion, carrots and celery. Cook, stirring, until the vegetables begin to soften, 6 to 8 minutes. Add bell pepper, garlic, Italian seasoning, pepper and salt and cook, stirring, for 2 minutes.

2. Add broth, cabbage and tomato; increase heat to medium-high and bring to a boil. Reduce heat to maintain a simmer, partially cover and cook until all the vegetables are tender, 15 to 20 minutes more. Remove from heat and stir in vinegar.

Vegan Superfood Grain Bowls

INGREDIENTS

- 1 (8 ounce) pouch microwavable quinoa

- ½ cup hummus

- 2 tablespoons lemon juice

- 1 (5 ounce) package baby kale

- 1 (8 ounce) package refrigerated cooked whole baby beets, sliced (or 2 cups from salad bar)

- 1 cup frozen shelled edamame, thawed

- 1 medium avocado, sliced

- ¼ cup unsalted toasted sunflower seeds

INSTRUCTIONS

1. Prepare quinoa according to package Directions; set aside to cool.

2. Combine hummus and lemon juice in a small bowl. Thin with water to desired dressing consistency. Divide the dressing among 4 small condiment containers with lids and refrigerate.

3. Divide baby kale among 4 single-serving containers with lids. Top each with 1/2 cup of the quinoa, 1/2 cup beets, 1/4 cup edamame and 1 tablespoon sunflower seeds.

4. When ready to eat, top with 1/4 avocado and the hummus dressing.

NOURISHING GLUTEN-FREE VEGAN DINNER RECIPE IDEAS

Roasted Vegetable & Black Bean Tacos

INGREDIENTS

• 1 cup roasted root vegetables

• ½ cup cooked or canned black beans, rinsed

• 2 teaspoons extra-virgin olive oil

• 1 teaspoon ground cumin

• 1 teaspoon chili powder

• ½ teaspoon ground coriander

• ¼ teaspoon kosher salt

- ¼ teaspoon ground pepper

- 4 corn tortillas, lightly toasted or warmed

- ½ avocado, cut into 8 slices

- 1 lime, cut into wedges

- Chopped fresh cilantro & salsa for garnish

INSTRUCTIONS

1. Combine roasted root vegetables, beans, oil, cumin, chili powder, coriander, salt and pepper in a saucepan. Cover and cook over medium-low heat until heated through, 6 to 8 minutes.

2. Divide the mixture among the tortillas. Top with avocado. Serve with lime wedges. Garnish with cilantro and/or salsa, if desired.

Vegan White Bean Chili

INGREDIENTS

- ¼ cup avocado oil or canola oil

- 2 cups chopped seeded Anaheim or poblano chiles (about 3)

- 1 large onion, chopped

- 4 cloves garlic, minced

- ½ cup quinoa, rinsed

- 4 teaspoons dried oregano

- 4 teaspoons ground cumin

- 1 teaspoon salt

- ½ teaspoon ground coriander

• ½ teaspoon ground pepper

• 4 cups low-sodium vegetable broth

• 2 (15 ounce) cans no-salt-added white beans, rinsed

• 1 large zucchini, diced (about 3 cups)

• ¼ cup chopped fresh cilantro

• 2 tablespoons lime juice, plus wedges for serving

INSTRUCTIONS

1. Heat oil in a large pot over medium heat. Add chiles, onion and garlic. Cook, stirring, until the vegetables are softened, 5 to 7 minutes. Add quinoa, oregano, cumin, salt, coriander and pepper; cook, stirring, until aromatic, about 1 minute. Stir in broth and beans. Bring to a boil. Reduce heat to a simmer. Partially cover and cook, stirring occasionally, for

20 minutes. Add zucchini; cover and continue cooking until the zucchini is soft and the chili has thickened, 10 to 15 minutes more. Stir in cilantro and lime juice. Serve with lime wedges, if desired.

No-Cook Black Bean Salad

INGREDIENTS

• ½ cup thinly sliced red onion

• 1 medium ripe avocado, pitted and roughly chopped

• ¼ cup cilantro leaves

• ¼ cup lime juice

• 2 tablespoons extra-virgin olive oil

• 1 clove garlic, minced

• ½ teaspoon salt

• 8 cups mixed salad greens

• 2 medium ears corn, kernels removed, or 2 cups frozen corn, thawed and patted dry

• 1 pint grape tomatoes, halved

• 1 (15 ounce) can black beans, rinsed

INSTRUCTIONS

1. Place onion in a medium bowl and cover with cold water. Set aside. Combine avocado, cilantro, lime juice, oil, garlic and salt in a mini food processor. Process, scraping down the sides as needed, until smooth and creamy.

2. Just before serving, combine salad greens, corn, tomatoes and beans in a large bowl. Drain the

onions and add to the bowl, along with the avocado dressing. Toss to coat.

Stuffed Sweet Potato with Hummus Dressing

INGREDIENTS

• 1 large sweet potato, scrubbed

• ¾ cup chopped kale

• 1 cup canned black beans, rinsed

• ¼ cup hummus

• 2 tablespoons water

INSTRUCTIONS

1. Prick sweet potato all over with a fork. Microwave on High until cooked through, 7 to 10 minutes.

2. Meanwhile, wash kale and drain, allowing water to cling to the leaves. Place in a medium saucepan; cover and cook over medium-high heat, stirring once or twice, until wilted. Add beans; add a tablespoon or two of water if the pot is dry. Continue cooking, uncovered, stirring occasionally, until the mixture is steaming hot, 1 to 2 minutes.

3. Split the sweet potato open and top with the kale and bean mixture. Combine hummus and 2 tablespoons water in a small dish. Add additional water as needed to reach desired consistency. Drizzle the hummus dressing over the stuffed sweet potato.

Chickpea & Quinoa Grain Bowl

INGREDIENTS

• 1 cup cooked quinoa

- ⅓ cup canned chickpeas, rinsed and drained

- ½ cup cucumber slices

- ½ cup cherry tomatoes, halved

- ¼ avocado, diced

- 3 tablespoons hummus

- 1 tablespoon finely chopped roasted red pepper

- 1 tablespoon lemon juice

- 1 tablespoon water, plus more if desired

- 1 teaspoon chopped fresh parsley (Optional)

- Pinch of salt

- Pinch of ground pepper

INSTRUCTIONS

1. Arrange quinoa, chickpeas, cucumbers, tomatoes and avocado in a wide bowl.

2. Stir hummus, roasted red pepper, lemon juice and water in a bowl. Add more water to reach desired consistency for dressing. Add parsley, salt and pepper and stir to combine. Serve with the grain bowl.

Chickpea Pasta with Mushrooms & Kale

INGREDIENTS

• 8 ounces chickpea rotini or penne (see Tip)

• ¼ cup extra-virgin olive oil

• 2 large cloves garlic, sliced

• Pinch of crushed red pepper

• 8 cups chopped kale

• 8 ounces cremini mushrooms, quartered

• ½ teaspoon dried thyme

• ½ teaspoon salt

• Grated Parmesan cheese for serving (optional)

INSTRUCTIONS

1. Cook pasta according to package Directions. Reserve 1 cup of the cooking water, then drain.

2. Meanwhile, heat oil in a large skillet over medium heat. Add garlic and crushed red pepper; cook, stirring once, until fragrant, about 1 minute. Add kale, mushrooms, thyme and salt; cook, stirring occasionally, until the vegetables are soft, about 5 minutes.

3. Stir in the pasta and enough of the reserved water to coat; cook, stirring, until combined and hot,

about 1 minute more. Serve topped with Parmesan, if desired.

Tip:

We chose chickpea pasta for this dish instead of whole-wheat because it's packed with tons of fiber, protein and nutrients—some brands provide more than 40% of your daily recommended fiber, plus 20 grams of protein per serving. Look for it with other gluten-free pastas.

Red Lentil Soup with Saffron

INGREDIENTS

• 3 tablespoons extra-virgin olive oil

• 2 medium carrots, finely diced

• 2 stalks celery, finely diced

• 1 large onion, finely diced

• 3 cloves garlic, minced

• 1 tablespoon tomato paste

• ½ teaspoon ground cumin

• ¼ teaspoon crushed saffron threads

• ¼ teaspoon ground turmeric

• 4 cups low-sodium no-chicken or chicken broth

• 1 ½ cups water, plus more as needed

• 1 pound red lentils (2 cups), picked over and rinsed

• 5 ounces spinach, coarsely chopped

• 1 teaspoon kosher salt

• 1 teaspoon ground pepper

• Plain yogurt & chopped fresh mint for garnish

INSTRUCTIONS

1. Heat oil in a large heavy pot over medium heat. Add carrots, celery and onion and cook until starting to soften, 7 to 10 minutes. (Do not brown.) Stir in garlic, tomato paste, cumin, saffron and turmeric and cook for 1 minute.

2. Add broth, water, lentils, spinach, salt and pepper. Bring to a simmer. Adjust heat to maintain a simmer, cover and cook, stirring as needed to prevent sticking, until the lentils and vegetables are tender, 15 to 20 minutes. Add more water if desired.

3. Garnish with yogurt and mint, if desired.

Quinoa, Avocado & Chickpea Salad over Mixed Greens

INGREDIENTS

• ⅔ cup water

• ⅓ cup quinoa

• ¼ teaspoon kosher salt or other coarse salt

• 1 clove garlic, crushed and peeled

• 2 teaspoons grated lemon zest

• 3 tablespoons lemon juice

• 3 tablespoons olive oil

• ¼ teaspoon ground pepper

• 1 cup rinsed no-salt-added canned chickpeas

• 1 medium carrot, shredded (1/2 cup)

• ½ avocado, diced

• 1 (5 ounce) package prewashed mixed greens, such as spring mix or baby kale-spinach blend (8 cups packed)

INSTRUCTIONS

1. Bring water to a boil in a small saucepan. Stir in quinoa. Reduce heat to low, cover, and simmer until all the liquid is absorbed, about 15 minutes. Use a fork to fluff and separate the grains; let cool for 5 minutes.

2. Meanwhile, sprinkle salt over garlic on a cutting board. Mash the garlic with the side of a spoon until a paste forms. Scrape into a medium bowl. Whisk in lemon zest, lemon juice, oil, and pepper. Transfer 3 Tbsp. of the dressing to a small bowl and set aside.

3. Add chickpeas, carrot, and avocado to the bowl with the remaining dressing; gently toss to combine. Let stand for 5 minutes to allow flavors to blend. Add the quinoa and gently toss to coat.

4. Place greens in a large bowl and toss with the reserved 3 Tbsp. dressing. Divide the greens between 2 plates and top with the quinoa mixture.

Four-Bean & Pumpkin Chili

INGREDIENTS

• 1 tablespoon extra-virgin olive oil

• 3 cups chopped onion

• 1 ½ cups chopped carrot

• 3 large cloves garlic, minced

• 4 cups low-sodium vegetable broth

• 3 cups diced pumpkin or butternut squash

• 1 (28 ounce) can no-salt-added crushed tomatoes

• 4 (15 ounce) cans low-sodium beans, such as black, great northern, pinto and/or red, rinsed

• 3 tablespoons chili powder

• 2 teaspoons ground cumin

• 1 teaspoon ground cinnamon

• ¾ teaspoon salt

• ¼ teaspoon cayenne pepper, or to taste

• Diced onion, sliced jalapeños, Cotija cheese and/or pepitas for garnish

INSTRUCTIONS

1. Heat oil in a large pot over medium-high heat. Add onion and cook, stirring often, until starting to

brown, about 5 minutes. Reduce heat to medium, add carrot and continue cooking, stirring often, until the vegetables are soft, 4 to 5 minutes more. Add garlic and cook, stirring, for 1 minute.

2. Stir in broth, scraping up any browned bits, and bring to a boil over high heat. Add pumpkin (or squash), tomatoes, beans, chili powder, cumin, cinnamon, salt and cayenne (if using). Cover and return to a boil. Reduce heat to maintain a gentle simmer and cook, uncovered, until the pumpkin (or squash) is tender, about 30 minutes.

3. Serve garnished with onion, jalapeños, cheese and/or pepitas, if desired.

Tofu Tacos

INGREDIENTS

• 1 tablespoon chili powder

• 1 teaspoon ground cumin

• ½ teaspoon dried oregano

• ½ teaspoon salt

• ¼ teaspoon ground pepper

• ⅛ teaspoon ground cinnamon

• 1 (14 to 16 ounce) block extra-firm tofu, patted dry and cut into 1/2-inch pieces

• 3 tablespoons extra-virgin olive oil, divided

• ½ cup chopped onion

• 2 large cloves garlic, minced

• 1 (15 ounce) can black beans, rinsed

• 2 teaspoons cider vinegar

- ½ cup chopped cilantro

- 8 corn tortillas, warmed

- ¼ cup Shredded cabbage, pico de gallo and/or guacamole

INSTRUCTIONS

1. Combine chili powder, cumin, oregano, salt, pepper and cinnamon in a medium bowl. Add tofu and toss to coat. Set aside.

2. Heat 2 tablespoons oil in a large nonstick skillet over medium heat. Add onion; cook, stirring, until starting to soften, about 3 minutes. Add garlic; cook, stirring, for 1 minute. Increase heat to medium-high and add tofu; cook, stirring occasionally, until starting to brown, about 10 minutes. Add beans; cook, stirring, until heated through, 2 to 3 minutes. Remove from heat; stir in vinegar and cilantro.

3. To serve, fill each tortilla with about 1/3 cup tofu filling. Top with cabbage, pico de gallo and/or guacamole, if desired.

Spinach Salad with Roasted Sweet Potatoes, White Beans & Basil

INGREDIENTS

• 1 sweet potato (12 ounces), peeled and diced (1/2-inch)

• 5 tablespoons extra-virgin olive oil, divided

• ½ teaspoon ground pepper, divided

• ¼ teaspoon salt, divided

• ½ cup packed fresh basil leaves

• 3 tablespoons cider vinegar

- 1 tablespoon finely chopped shallot

- 2 teaspoons whole-grain mustard

- 10 cups baby spinach

- 1 (15 ounce) can low-sodium cannellini beans, rinsed

- 2 cups shredded cabbage

- 1 cup chopped red bell pepper

- ⅓ cup chopped pecans, toasted

INSTRUCTIONS

1. Preheat oven to 425 degrees F.

2. Toss sweet potatoes, 1 tablespoon oil, 1/4 teaspoon pepper and 1/8 teaspoon salt together in a large bowl. Transfer to a large rimmed baking sheet

and roast, stirring once, until tender, 15 to 18 minutes. Let cool for at least 10 minutes.

3. Meanwhile, place basil, the remaining 1/4 cup oil, vinegar, shallot, mustard and the remaining 1/4 teaspoon pepper and 1/8 teaspoon salt in a mini food processor. Process until mostly smooth. Transfer to the large bowl. Add spinach, beans, cabbage, bell pepper, pecans and the cooled sweet potatoes. Toss to coat.

Vegan Burrito Bowls with Cauliflower Rice

INGREDIENTS

• 1 recipe Tofu Crumbles

• 1 (12 ounce) package frozen riced cauliflower

• 4 teaspoons olive oil

- 1 teaspoon no-salt-added taco seasoning

- 1 cup thinly sliced red cabbage

- 1 cup diced avocado

- ½ cup pico de gallo or salsa

- ¼ cup chopped fresh cilantro

INSTRUCTIONS

1. Prepare Tofu Crumbles as directed.

2. While the Tofu Crumbles cook, prepare riced cauliflower according to package Directions. Toss with oil and taco seasoning.

3. Divide the cauliflower among 4 single-serving containers with lids. Top each with 1/2 cup Tofu Crumbles, 1/4 cup each cabbage and avocado, 2 tablespoons pico de gallo (or salsa) and 1 tablespoon

cilantro. Seal the containers and refrigerate until ready to eat.

Mushroom & Tofu Stir-Fry

INGREDIENTS

• 4 tablespoons peanut oil or canola oil, divided

• 1 pound mixed mushrooms, sliced

• 1 medium red bell pepper, diced

• 1 bunch scallions, trimmed and cut into 2-inch pieces

• 1 tablespoon grated fresh ginger

• 1 large clove garlic, grated

• 1 (8 ounce) container baked tofu or smoked tofu, diced

• 3 tablespoons oyster sauce or vegetarian oyster sauce (see Tip)

INSTRUCTIONS

1. Heat 2 tablespoons oil in a large flat-bottom wok or cast-iron skillet over high heat. Add mushrooms and bell pepper; cook, stirring occasionally, until soft, about 4 minutes. Stir in scallions, ginger and garlic; cook for 30 seconds more. Transfer the vegetables to a bowl.

2. Add the remaining 2 tablespoons oil and tofu to the pan. Cook, turning once, until browned, 3 to 4 minutes. Stir in the vegetables and oyster sauce. Cook, stirring, until hot, about 1 minute.

Tips

Tip: Sweet, salty oyster sauce is made from, well, oysters, along with salt, sugar and sometimes soy sauce. Substitute vegetarian oyster or stir-fry sauce, if desired, which uses mushrooms instead of oysters.

Grilled Eggplant Salad

INGREDIENTS

• ¼ cup olive oil

• 2 teaspoons za'atar (see Tips)

• 1 teaspoon lemon zest, plus 3 tablespoons lemon juice (from 1 lemon), divided

• 1 medium eggplant (about 1 pound), cut into 1/2-inch-thick slices

• 1 medium red bell pepper, stemmed, seeded and quartered lengthwise

• ½ medium red onion, peeled and cut into 1-inch wedges through the root

- Cooking spray

- 1 cup halved cherry tomatoes

- ¾ cup coarsely chopped fresh flat-leaf parsley

- ¼ cup thinly sliced scallions

- ¼ cup coarsely chopped fresh mint

- ½ teaspoon salt

INSTRUCTIONS

1. Preheat a grill to medium-high.

2. Combine oil, za'atar and lemon zest in a small bowl. Brush 1 side of eggplant slices with half of the oil mixture; reserve the remaining mixture. Oil the grill rack (see Tips). Grill the eggplant, uncovered, turning often, until tender and grill marks appear on both sides, about 5 minutes total. Cut the

eggplant into 1/4-inch pieces and transfer to a large bowl.

3. Coat bell pepper quarters and onion wedges with cooking spray. Grill, uncovered, until tender and charred, about 5 minutes. Chop the peppers into 3/4-inch pieces. Remove and discard onion stem. Add the peppers, onions, tomatoes, parsley, scallions and mint to the bowl with the eggplant.

4. Add lemon juice and salt to the reserved oil mixture; whisk to combine. Drizzle over the vegetables and toss to coat.

Tips

Tips: The Middle Eastern spice blend za'atar gives you big flavor from just one ingredient: it's a mix of thyme, sumac, salt, sesame seeds and sometimes other herbs. Look for it in the bulk-spice section of natural-foods stores, in specialty-foods stores, in the spice section of some grocery stores or online. To make your own mix: Combine 1 tsp. each ground sumac, sesame seeds and dried thyme with 1/4 tsp. salt.

To oil a grill rack, oil a folded paper towel, hold it with tongs and rub it over the rack. (Do not use cooking spray on a hot grill.)

Thai Coconut Curry Soup

INGREDIENTS

• 6 cups low-sodium vegetable broth, divided

• ¾ ounce dried shiitake mushrooms

• 1 tablespoon extra-virgin olive oil

• 1 ½ cups chopped onion

• 2 teaspoons grated fresh ginger

- 2 jalapeño peppers, minced

- 1 ½ tablespoons Thai red curry paste

- 1 ½ tablespoons reduced-sodium tamari

- 1 ½ teaspoons lime zest

- ¼ cup lime juice

- ½ teaspoon salt

- 2 ¼ cups coconut milk

- 12 ounces diced extra-firm tofu (1/2-inch)

- 3 ounces fresh oyster mushrooms or other wild mushrooms, chopped

- 4 cups chopped mature spinach (5 ounces)

- Fresh cilantro for garnish

INSTRUCTIONS

1. Combine 1 cup broth and dried shiitakes in a small saucepan. Bring to a boil over medium-high heat. Cover, reduce heat to maintain a simmer and cook for 10 minutes. Strain the broth through a coffee filter (or a double layer of cheesecloth) to catch the grit, and squeeze the mushrooms to extract as much liquid as possible. Reserve the cooking liquid and chop the mushrooms.

2. Meanwhile, heat oil in a large pot over medium-high heat. Add onion and cook, stirring frequently, until starting to brown, 2 to 4 minutes. Reduce heat to medium and continue cooking, stirring often, until the onion is soft, 3 to 5 minutes. Stir in the remaining 5 cups broth, scraping up any browned bits. Cover and bring to a boil over high heat. Add ginger, jalapeños, curry paste, tamari, lime zest and juice, salt and the reserved mushroom-cooking liquid. Cover and return to a boil.

3. Reduce heat to medium and add coconut milk, tofu, fresh mushrooms and the soaked shiitakes; return to a simmer and cook, partially covered, until the mushrooms are tender, 3 to 5 minutes. Stir in spinach and cook until wilted, 2 to 3 minutes more. Serve garnished with cilantro, if desired.

Tips

To make ahead: Refrigerate for up to 5 days.

GLUTEN-FREE VEGAN RECIPES FOR SNACKS AND DESSERTS

Pink Lemonade Nice Cream

INGREDIENTS

• 3 medium ripe bananas, sliced and frozen

• ⅔ cup fresh or frozen raspberries

• 1 tablespoon lemon zest

• 2 tablespoons lemon juice

INSTRUCTIONS

1. Place bananas, raspberries, lemon zest and lemon juice in a food processor. Process until smooth.

No-Sugar-Added Vegan Oatmeal Cookies

INGREDIENTS

- 1 cup quick-cooking oats (see Tip)

- ¾ cup almond flour or almond meal

- ¾ teaspoon ground cinnamon

- ¼ teaspoon salt

- 2 medium ripe bananas, mashed

- ½ cup almond butter or natural peanut butter

- 1 teaspoon vanilla extract

- ¾ cup raisins or chopped dates

INSTRUCTIONS

1. Preheat oven to 350 degrees F. Line a large baking sheet with parchment paper or a silicone baking mat.

2. Whisk oats, almond flour (or almond meal), cinnamon and salt in a medium bowl. Mash bananas, almond butter (or peanut butter) and vanilla together in a large bowl until creamy and well combined. Add the dry ingredients and raisins (or dates) to the banana mixture and stir with a wooden spoon until combined. Scoop or roll level tablespoons of dough into balls and place on the prepared baking sheet, making 12 cookies per batch. Press with a fork to flatten slightly.

3. Bake until firm to the touch and light brown on the bottom, about 15 minutes. Transfer to a wire rack to cool completely. Repeat with the remaining batter.

Tips

Tip: People with celiac disease or gluten sensitivity should use oats that are labeled "gluten-free," as oats are often cross-contaminated with wheat and barley.

Pineapple Nice Cream

INGREDIENTS

• 1 16-ounce package frozen pineapple chunks

• 1 cup frozen mango chunks or 1 large mango, peeled, seeded and chopped

• 1 tablespoon lemon juice or lime juice

INSTRUCTIONS

1. Process pineapple, mango and lemon (or lime) juice in a food processor until smooth and creamy. (If using frozen mango, you may have to add up to

1/4 cup water.) For the best texture, serve immediately.

Virgin Banana Piña Colada Pops

INGREDIENTS

• 2 very ripe bananas, sliced

• 1 cup diced fresh pineapple

• 1 cup pineapple juice

• 1 cup coconut milk (see Tip)

INSTRUCTIONS

1. Combine bananas, pineapple, pineapple juice and coconut milk in a blender. Puree until smooth. Divide among ten 3-ounce popsicle molds and freeze until firm, at least 4 hours.

Tips

To make ahead: Freeze for up to 3 weeks.

Equipment: Ten 3-ounce (or similar-size) freezer-pop molds

Tip: Shake the can of coconut milk well before using. Refrigerate leftover coconut milk for up to 1 week or freeze for up to 2 months. It will appear separated when thawed; simply mix until smooth.

Apple "Donuts"

INGREDIENTS

• 1 medium apple

• 3 tablespoons almond butter

• 2 teaspoons shredded unsweetened coconut

INSTRUCTIONS

1. Remove apple core with an apple coring tool. Slice the apple crosswise into 8 thin rings, about 1/4 inch thick. Spread each apple ring with almond butter. Sprinkle with coconut.

Chunky Peach Popsicles

INGREDIENTS

• 1 1/4 pounds ripe peaches, (3-4 medium), halved and pitted

• Juice of 1 lemon

• ¼ cup freshly squeezed orange juice

• ¼ cup sugar, or to taste

• ¼ teaspoon vanilla extract

1. Coarsely chop peaches in a food processor. Transfer 1 cup of the chunky peaches to a medium bowl. Add lemon juice, orange juice and sugar to taste (depending on the sweetness of the peaches) to the food processor. Puree until smooth. Add to the bowl with the chunky peaches and stir in vanilla.

2. Divide the mixture among twelve 2-ounce or eight 3-ounce freezer-pop molds (or small paper cups). Freeze until beginning to set, about 1 hour. Insert frozen-treat sticks and freeze until completely firm, about 1 hour more.

Frozen Chocolate-Coconut Milk with Strawberries

INGREDIENTS

• ½ cup nondairy chocolate-coconut frozen dessert

• 8 medium strawberries, hulled and quartered

INSTRUCTIONS

1. Serve chocolate-coconut frozen dessert with strawberries.

Strawberry Nice Cream

INGREDIENTS

• 1 pound fresh strawberries

• 2 medium bananas

• 1 tablespoon fresh lemon juice

• ¼ cup ice-cold water, as needed

INSTRUCTIONS

1. Hull and coarsely chop strawberries. Peel and coarsely chop bananas. Spread the strawberries and bananas on separate sides of one baking sheet or on two sheets. Freeze until solid, at least 12 hours.

2. Let the strawberries thaw at room temperature for 15 minutes. Transfer to a food processor; pulse until finely chopped, about 10 pulses. Add the frozen bananas and lemon juice; process until smooth, 1 to 1 1/2 minutes, adding up to 1/4 cup cold water if needed to achieve desired consistency, stopping to scrape down sides of bowl as needed. Serve immediately or, for a firmer texture, transfer to a freezer-safe container and freeze for up to 30 minutes.

"Chocomole" Pudding

INGREDIENTS

- 16 Medjool dates, pitted and coarsely chopped

- 3 ripe avocados

- 1 cup unsweetened almond milk or coconut milk beverage

- 1 cup unsweetened cocoa powder

- ¼ cup pure maple syrup or agave nectar

- 1 tablespoon coconut oil

- 1 teaspoon vanilla extract

- Pinch of sea salt, plus more for garnish

INSTRUCTIONS

1. Soak dates in 1 cup hot water until soft, 5 to 10 minutes. Drain.

2. Process the dates, avocados, milk beverage, cocoa, maple syrup (or agave), oil, vanilla and a

pinch of salt in a food processor until very smooth and creamy. Refrigerate until cold, about 3 hours. Serve garnished with a little extra sea salt, if desired.

Vegan No-Bake Cookies

INGREDIENTS

• ¾ cup almond butter or natural peanut butter

• ⅓ cup packed brown sugar (light or dark)

• ¼ cup coconut oil

• ¼ cup unsweetened almond milk

• 1 ¾ cups rolled oats (see Tip)

• 1 teaspoon ground cinnamon

• 1 teaspoon vanilla extract

• ⅛ teaspoon salt

INSTRUCTIONS

1. Heat almond butter (or peanut butter), brown sugar, coconut oil and almond milk in a medium saucepan over medium heat, stirring, until the oil and sugar have melted. Stir in oats, cinnamon, vanilla and salt. Let cool slightly.

2. Drop the dough by tablespoonfuls onto a parchment-lined baking sheet. Press into 2-inch circles. Refrigerate until firm, about 2 hours.

Tips

To make ahead: Refrigerate in an airtight container for up to 5 days.

Tip: People with celiac disease or gluten sensitivity should use oats that are labeled "gluten-free," as oats are often cross-contaminated with wheat and barley.

Dairy-Free Banana Rice Pudding

INGREDIENTS

- 1 cup brown basmati rice

- 2 cups water

- ½ teaspoon salt

- 3 cups plus 1 tablespoon gluten-free vanilla rice milk, divided (see Tip)

- ⅓ cup light brown sugar

- ½ teaspoon ground cinnamon, plus more for garnish

- 1 tablespoon cornstarch

- 4 ripe bananas, divided

- 1 teaspoon vanilla extract

INSTRUCTIONS

1. Combine rice, water and salt in a medium saucepan and bring to a boil. Reduce heat to low, cover and cook until the liquid is fully absorbed, 45 to 50 minutes.

2. Stir in 3 cups rice milk, brown sugar and 1/2 teaspoon cinnamon and bring to a lively simmer. Cook, stirring occasionally, for 10 minutes. Stir cornstarch and the remaining 1 tablespoon rice milk in a small bowl until smooth; add to the pudding. Continue cooking, stirring often, until the mixture is the consistency of porridge, about 10 minutes. Remove from the heat.

3. Mash 2 bananas in a small bowl. Stir the mashed bananas and vanilla into the pudding. Transfer to a large bowl, press plastic wrap directly onto the surface of the pudding and refrigerate until cold, at least 2 hours.

4. Just before serving, slice the remaining 2 bananas. Top each serving with a few slices of banana and sprinkle with cinnamon, if desired.

Tips

Make Ahead Tip: Prepare through Step 3, cover and refrigerate for up to 1 day. Finish with Step 4 just before serving.

Tip: Some brands of rice milk may contain gluten. Gluten-free brands include Pacific Natural Foods or 365 Organic.

2-Ingredient Peanut Butter Banana Ice Cream

INGREDIENTS

• 2 medium bananas, peeled, halved and frozen

• ¼ cup natural peanut butter

• Unsweetened shredded coconut for garnish

INSTRUCTIONS

1. Place bananas and peanut butter in a food processor. Pulse and process until mostly smooth, stopping to scrape down the sides as needed. Garnish with coconut, if desired. Serve immediately.

Crispy Peanut Butter Balls

INGREDIENTS

• ½ cup natural peanut butter, almond butter or sunflower seed butter

• ¾ cup crispy rice cereal

• 1 teaspoon pure maple syrup

• ½ cup dark chocolate chips, melted (see Tip)

INSTRUCTIONS

1. Line a baking sheet with parchment or wax paper. Combine peanut butter, cereal and maple syrup in a medium bowl. Roll the mixture into 12 balls, using about 2 teaspoons for each. Place on the prepared baking sheet. Freeze the balls until firm, about 15 minutes.

2. Roll the balls in melted chocolate. Return to the freezer until the chocolate is set, about 15 minutes.

Tips

To make ahead: Refrigerate in an airtight container for up to 3 weeks.

Tip: To melt chocolate, microwave on Medium for 1 minute. Stir, then continue microwaving on Medium, stirring every 20 seconds, until melted. Or place chocolate in the top of a double boiler over hot, but not boiling, water. Stir until melted.

Strawberry-Mango Nice Cream

INGREDIENTS

• 12 ounces frozen mango chunks

• 8 ounces frozen sliced strawberries

• 1 tablespoon lime juice

INSTRUCTIONS

1. Place mango, strawberries and lime juice in a food processor; process for 1 to 2 minutes. Stop the processor and scrape down the sides. Continue processing until smooth, an additional 2 to 3 minutes, adding up to 1/2 cup water to help process the fruit, if necessary.

Tips

To make ahead: While the nice cream will have the best texture if served immediately, it can be stored in the freezer for up to 3 months. Allow it to soften at room temperature for about an hour before serving.

CHAPTER VI

TO SUM UP

Adopting a gluten-free vegan diet presents a unique intersection of health considerations, ethical values, and dietary needs. For those with celiac disease or gluten sensitivity, the elimination of gluten is a non-negotiable aspect of their dietary regimen, crucial for avoiding adverse health reactions and maintaining overall well-being. Coupled with veganism—a lifestyle choice driven by a commitment to animal welfare, environmental sustainability, and personal health—this dietary combination can pose both opportunities and challenges.

One of the primary benefits of a gluten-free vegan diet is its potential to promote a heightened awareness of food choices. Individuals who adhere to this diet often find themselves more attuned to the ingredients and nutritional profiles of their meals, which can lead to a greater emphasis on whole, unprocessed foods. This mindfulness can be advantageous, fostering a diet rich in fruits, vegetables, legumes, nuts, and seeds. Such a diet is typically high in essential vitamins, minerals, and antioxidants while being low in saturated fats and cholesterol, potentially supporting long-term cardiovascular health and overall vitality.

However, the journey to maintaining a balanced gluten-free vegan diet is not without its difficulties. Ensuring adequate intake of certain nutrients can be a complex endeavor. Nutrients such as vitamin B12, iron, calcium, and omega-3 fatty acids are often found in animal products or gluten-containing grains, necessitating careful planning and, in some cases, supplementation. The reliance on fortified foods and supplements must be thoughtfully managed to avoid deficiencies and ensure nutritional adequacy.

 Moreover, the social and cultural aspects of eating can also pose challenges. Dining out or participating in social gatherings may require advanced planning and communication, as many restaurants and social events may not readily accommodate the specific requirements of a gluten-free vegan diet. This aspect can sometimes lead to a sense of isolation or inconvenience, underscoring the importance of finding supportive communities and resources.

Despite these challenges, many people find the commitment to a gluten-free vegan diet to be deeply rewarding. The alignment with personal values regarding animal welfare and environmental sustainability can provide a strong sense of purpose and satisfaction. Additionally, the increased focus on whole, plant-based foods often leads to a renewed appreciation for diverse culinary experiences and a deeper connection to the origins of one's food.

In summary, while a gluten-free vegan diet demands careful consideration and diligent effort, it offers a path to health and ethical living that resonates profoundly with many individuals. The key to success lies in informed planning, a willingness to adapt, and the continuous pursuit of balanced nutrition. Embracing this dietary approach can lead to a holistic sense of well-being, both physically and morally, reflecting a conscientious commitment to personal health and broader environmental and ethical principles.